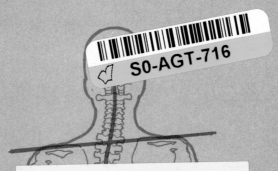

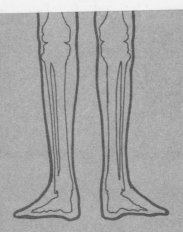

Ex Libris

Donna R. MacDonald

DR. THOMPSON'S
NEW WAY FOR
YOU TO CURE
YOUR ACHING
BACK

Books by Jess Stearn

Non-Fiction

Fiction

Jess Stearn

DR. THOMPSON'S NEW WAY FOR YOU TO CURE YOUR ACHING BACK

1973

Doubleday & Company, Inc., Garden City, New York

Endpapers by Helen Brennon

ISBN: 0-385-00473-7
Library of Congress Catalog Card Number 72-96260
Copyright © 1973 by Alec Thompson and Jess Stearn
Printed in the United States of America
First Edition

This book is dedicated to everyone who has ever
had a bad back.

CONTENTS

DR. THOMPSON'S
NEW WAY FOR
YOU TO CURE
———
YOUR ACHING
BACK

CHAPTER I   *An Introduction of Sorts*

Dr. Alec Thompson has helped thousands to repair their aching backs. I am one of the fortunates, and out of my own experience came the idea for a self-help book to help others who could not conveniently get help from the kindly capable physician of Westwood Village, Los Angeles. Without this friendly bear of a man, I would still be troubled with the aching back—and neck—that troubled me for years.

I had finally reconciled myself to the medical opinion that I would have to learn to live with it. After many treatments to correct a serious whiplash injury, I would feel relief for a while and then the old familiar soreness would be back. Along with the whiplash, as often happens with a severe automobile injury, my lower back was also giving me trouble, as the sacroiliac joint was constantly slipping out of joint. I felt an acute low backache, marked by stiffness when I sat for any time at my typewriter, in an airplane, at the wheel of my car.

But after only one visit to Dr. Thompson's office, I have had no more problem with my sacroiliac. For when the doctor got through with his spinal adjustment, he showed me how I could "adjust" my own hip, putting it into place just as easily and effectively as he had.

This spinal corrective exercise, along with certain other preventive and rejuvenating exercises, he considers his contribution to millions of back-sufferers with disc problems, sciatica, low-backache, abnormally curved or rounded spines. And the benefits from these exercises extend to even those people suffering from migraine headaches, premature aging, even sexual inadequacy.

The idea for Thompson's corrective exercise came in response to an obvious need. It was expensive and time-consuming for patients to trip back and forth to his office to have their backs straightened. And so Thompson came up one day with a corrective exercise designed to let the suffering traveler put his own aching back in place.

"It had to be something very simple, and effective, which the layman could do wherever he was," he observed.

It can be done sitting, standing, lying down, and it can be done by anybody who can put one hand around his ankle and another around his knee, angle the heel over the groin, and pull back evenly with both hands. It is so wonderfully simple that few, until they try it, believe it can almost surely relieve their aching back and their sciatica—being in effect a specific for both disorders.

I have done the exercise myself, and have seen it work on others. It is remarkably effective, and there is no chance of harming oneself. There is no strain or pressure, and there is little to remember in performing the exercise properly. Nevertheless, many people have had trouble getting the position down properly the first time, so it will be repeated throughout the book—and with other therapeutic exercises of a revitalizing nature diagramed in the appendix at the end of the book. For unless it is done correctly, the corrective exercise will have no result, favorable or unfavorable.

Dr. Thompson has a medical degree, but was trained in osteopathy, that part of medicine which believes that the body is a self-healing mechanism, ready to heal itself, given the chance.

Some might call it unconventional therapy, but it works.

I had my own experience with conventional therapy for a slipped sacroiliac at twenty-five. In retrospect, I realized that I had thrown myself out of joint in reaching for a suitcase in an overhead rack at a time when the train I was on suddenly decided to lurch. I felt first an ache in my right hip, then the left, as the unevenness of my walk, affected both sides. Then came shooting pains down my right leg, and after a week or so, I could hardly lift myself out of a chair or walk down the street without leaning against the side of a building.

I had gone to two doctors, and neither could help me. One had suggested rest, hot sitz baths, and an acid-free diet. I did all this, and the pain seemed to get worse. The second doctor recommended caudal surgery.

My back problem was becoming an emotional problem. How, I asked myself, could I stay on my job as a newspaper reporter and support a wife and small child? I had trouble getting to sleep, and when I did drop off, would wake up suddenly in a cold sweat.

When my mental state was lowest, destiny or chance came to my aid.

Still hobbling to work, I was assigned one day to do a feature article on the people who keep other people's bodies trim. My halting steps took me to New York City's Rockefeller Center, where the rich and the famous—the Eddie Rickenbackers, Bob Hopes, and General Sarnoffs—went to keep their aging bodies on a par with youthful minds. There, I met the personable proprietor, physiotherapist-chiropractor Harold J. Reilly, the epitome of the fitness he was espousing.

I was shown the various exercises and manipulative treatments that Reilly used, and was duly impressed by the finished products of indeterminate age who floated in and out of treatment rooms. Whether they were forty, fifty, sixty, even seventy, his people were vigorous and vital, full of themselves and their plans.

Having gathered my material, I was saying farewell to Reilly when his blue eyes twinkled back at me.

"Now that you've skirted the edges of the pool, why don't you jump in?"

"What do you mean?" I asked.

"A young fellow like you shouldn't be hobbling around like that," he said.

His eyes were now traveling over my lower spine.

"I would like to measure your legs."

He stretched me out on a table and brought out a tape measure.

"Just as I thought," he murmured. "Your legs measure the same length individually, but together one is an inch and a quarter shorter than the other. On this basis, I would say your sacroiliac is way out of joint."

"But I have sciatica," I protested.

He nodded good-naturedly. "But that's only the result, not the cause."

He asked me to relax comfortably on my back.

"If you have no objection," he said, "I'll slip that joint back in place."

He took hold of one leg by the ankle, and deftly brought the knee into my groin, then repeated the move with the other leg. I felt an immediate easing of pressure in my lower back. I stood up and tested my legs gingerly. There was no pain. The muscle spasm in my hip was still sensitive to my touch, but the pain down my leg had ceased.

He smiled. "Come back every two or three days for the next two weeks or so, as that adjustment will require a little reinforcing, since your hip has been displaced so long."

In two weeks, my hip was stabilized, and the pain had vanished. I walked, bent, twisted with new confidence. The specter of a lifelong bout with an agonizing ailment had ended thanks to this gifted therapist, who is still helping people at his new place in Oak Ridge, New Jersey.

Dr. Thompson had come along with a self-help procedure, when the public was readier to accept a therapy essentially mechanistic in nature.

I was constantly testing the Thompson do-it-yourself technique. There seemed no limit to the practical application of his postulation that the sacroiliac was the cause of bodily ills of nearly every variety. Jan Robinson, an associate of novelist Taylor Caldwell, had been complaining about a painful knob on her thumb impairing the usefulness of her hand. The doctor's eye went to her hand, and then traveled over her spine.

He asked her to stand up.

Plainly puzzled, Mrs. Robinson rose to her feet.

"It's my right hand that's bothering me," she stressed, "the thumb."

Thompson nodded absently, and touched her spine.

"You are the victim of a chain of events involving the right side, starting with the shoulder, then the elbow, and the hand and thumb. Obviously, there has been a nerve impairment, and this suggests a familiar pattern years in forming. The intensity of the connected injuries tells of harmful inflammatory changes. Instead of just looking at the hand itself, and the swelling around the thumb, I look for a basic source, the tributary nerve impulses which radiate to the arms and shoulders from the spine."

He cast a quizzical eye at Jan's spine. "Even through her clothing, we note that the left pelvic or hipbone is lower than the right at its crest, that some distance above there is a scoliotic or lateral curvature of the spine. And we know we are dealing with scoliotic stress."

He continued to trace her thumb problem—only a symptom, it now appeared—back to its source.

"It's a matter of understanding how your body works. There's a total relationship within the system, with the nerve flow from one area eventually affecting normal movements elsewhere. What bothers your toe may bother your eye. Every blood vessel in your body has a nerve with it, down to the tiniest capillary. Every muscle, every tissue, every ligament and tendon, has a neurological involvement. A nerve stimulus from the spine may affect certain areas within the viscera—the heart, liver, intestines, etc., and these in turn feed back their messages to the spine. You just can't have one thing wrong with you very long.

"Basically," he told Jan, "you reflect a stress in the lower cervical [neck vertebra] and upper dorsal area [upper back] affecting any nerve impulse from that area, and in turn, affecting the function of the right arm."

Jan now seemed thoroughly confused.

"Knowing that the thumb is only a result," he explained, "there is not much point to treating the thumb while not getting at the cause which is plainly related to the maladjustment at the base of the spine."

Jan and I anticipated a rigorous manipulative procedure to get her spine back in order.

Dr. Thompson gave me a grin.

"I see you don't believe in the spinal corrective exercise."

"You mean," I said almost incredulously, "that she can treat herself?"

He shrugged. "Why not? If it doesn't work for her, it won't work for anybody. And if it works for anybody, it works for her. The only problem is that she's had a displacement for years, so it will take a correspondingly longer time for her sacroiliac to stabilize itself, and in turn straighten out the spinal scoliosis which is affecting her right shoulder, arm, and thumb."

He gave her spine another critical look.

"What we do now is give her the proper exercise to correct the hipbones, correcting the obvious misalignment. This exercise, sufficiently repeated at first—every hour on the hour if she likes—will bring the tilted left sacroiliac joint back into its original position. As that stays in position and the ilial bones become evenly aligned for increasing periods, the sacral bone becomes firmly wedged between the two ilial bones, and forms a strong even base for the spinal column which rests on it. And with this base perfectly straight, there is no longer any need for the spine and its vertebra to tilt compensatingly, and it straightens out in its normal curve."

Just as the chain reaction had sprung damagingly from the sacroiliac to the upper spine to the shoulder and the arm, so he now intended to reverse the procedure. As much as I respected Dr. Thompson, it seemed hardly likely that a simple adjustment of the sacroiliac would eliminate the swelling in Jan Robinson's thumb.

Dr. Thompson's attention was still on his patient.

"Your first rib is also out of position," he said. "That would cause a definite pressure of the capsular ligament around the rib which affects the nerve involvement in that area."

He pressed authoritatively against the rib. I could hear it pop back in place.

"I'm just helping things along," he said. "It would return in time to its normal position, once the sacroiliac is in place."

He now had Jan lie down comfortably, and bring her

ankle and knee back in the corrective exercise he had shown her.

"You don't use any pressure, just bring both back easily and relax for a minute or so. Then do it with the other side. You have five years of misalignment to correct all at once."

After a couple of minutes, Jan got up and began walking around the living room.

"It may be my imagination," she said, "but I feel better already."

She put her hands on her hips.

"How about checking me out now?"

"The crest of the ilial bones looks level and I'd say you're on your way to getting rid of your scoliosis and your bad thumb. Just keep up the exercise."

"How often should I do it?" she asked.

"As often as you like—up to twenty times a day if you choose."

Jan Robinson was moving about, happy in her new-found freedom.

"How can you tell for sure that you're level?" she asked.

"First, by the way you feel," he replied. "There's an absence of pressure, a volatility of motion. And then by checking your pubic bones"—he pointed to the groin—"in a mirror. When the ilial or hipbones are properly lined up, the pubic bones are straight across from each other."

I wondered how common was this maladjustment of the sacroiliac and the pelvis it was part of.

"The sacroiliac can go out no matter your age or occupation. It doesn't matter whether you're two years old or a hundred. And the condition can persist ten, twenty, thirty years, with the victims never feeling right, constantly getting treatment for symptoms rather than causes, for backaches, armaches, headaches. They become weary from the endless tension in their joints and ligaments. The body is never free and relaxed. They strain every time they get up from a chair, and they are forever straining to accomplish with maximum effort what should be simply achieved."

"How come," Jan asked, "that nobody bothered to tell me that I had a curvature?"

"Nobody bothered to look. Everybody has a tendency to look at what pains a person, not at what causes the pain. You go into the average doctor's office, and you say, 'My hand hurts.' Is he going to look at your spine, your back, in relationship to your hand? No, he's going to look at your hand and say, 'Well, this thing is swollen. I guess we'll have to put something on it.' Or perhaps he'll advise shortwave diathermy, or some ultrasonic technique, anything to relieve the swelling. He may give you pills for the pain, some cold soaks or some hot soaks depending on whether he believes in cold or hot, and he may get that swelling down. But nothing is being done about what is actually causing the swelling."

He gave Jan a wry look. "I can treat your thumb locally but the swelling may come back again or there may be a nerve involvement eventually with another finger. Meanwhile, you find your arm getting weaker and weaker and pretty soon it may be an effort to pick up anything with this arm. And then you may go to a neurosurgeon, who will at least trace it back to the arm, and the spine, and he may even tell you that you have a disc that will have to come out in the cervical [upper spinal] area. But even so, you're still not getting at the cause, in the pelvic area."

Jan frowned. "Why didn't I notice this pelvic tilt myself? God knows I look at myself enough in the mirror."

Thompson laughed. "Women are used to looking in the mirror but curvatures are not what they're looking for. It is not hard to pick out. If you have any abdominal fat at all, looking in the mirror closely you'll find if you have scoliotic curvature there will be multiple folds on one side in comparison to the other side. Maybe if we all ran around three quarters nude and got to know what we really looked like, it would keep us from middle-age sag and other debilities. We just couldn't stand looking at ourselves."

The session with Jan Robinson had taken but a few minutes. As she said goodbye and the door closed on her, Dr. Thompson sighed unhappily.

"I am not sure I convinced her that her real problem is in the lower back."

The doctor should not have worried. A month later, in Mrs. Robinson's native Buffalo, when I saw her again, she held up her right thumb triumphantly.

"Look," she said, "the swelling is gone."

I did not have to ask whether she had done the corrective exercise.

And now, for a more intimate presentation of his exercises, Dr. Thompson's experience with patients is described hereafter by him in the first person singular.

CHAPTER II

Dr. Thompson Discusses: Anatomy of a Backache

You are bending to the floor, picking up a spoon, a button, a needle, a pin. You start to straighten up, as you have a hundred times before. Suddenly, there is an unexpected twinge in the lumbar, lower back, area. The pain may start shooting down one leg, circling the hip or waist and traveling up the spine. If you look at a mirror, you can see that your trunk is tilted. No matter how you try, you can't bring yourself up straight. Your muscles are in spasm, and you are in trouble. Without any warning you have become a full-fledged member of a vast army of low-back casualties. And your problems may only be starting. You may be in for a period of discomfort, distress, and painfully restricted movement that could continue the rest of your life.

It may be a new, or an old, back problem. If old, then you are familiar with the many treatments that bring only temporary relief—traction, heat, massage, manipulation, pain killers, muscle relaxants, liniments.

What happened to you could have happened to any-

one at any time who is not in the peak of physical condition. And very few people, even professional athletes,
are in this condition without a special exercise routine
to keep the muscles, ligaments, and joints strong and
supple. In this case, something went wrong with the
sacroiliac. In trying to straighten up, your hipbones didn't
go along with the rest of you. The ligaments became overextended, pulling the ilium—hipbone—from its juncture
with the V-shaped sacrum at the base of the spine, and
causing the whole pelvic girdle—sacrum, hipbone, pubic bone—to painfully tilt.

The sacroiliac syndrome is all too familiar. In its acute
stage, as victims try to stand up, they may have to push
themselves up from the bed or chair. They are so stiff in
the morning they can hardly bend over. They reach over
to brush their teeth and their back almost kills them. When
the condition continues uncorrected, fibrous tissues become chronically inflamed and a lateral curvature or
scoliosis of the spine develops. These damaged tissues
are susceptible to temperature and moisture, and after
a while the individual often feels a dull ache that lets him
know rain is in the air.

When somebody comes in with a back problem, I have
learned to first check out the lower back for a sacroiliac
slippage. And invariably I find a displacement, even if it is
only slight and on but one side. Unless this slippage, with
its pelvic tilt, is corrected in time, the downward pressure of the scoliotic spinal column unevenly grinds down
the cushioned cartilage or discs between the vertebrae,
and may lead to a so-called disc problem. I seldom see
a total displacement of the sacroiliac. In automobile

accidents where ligaments are severely stretched, one leg could be as much as an inch and a half shorter or longer than the other yet the sacroiliac is not out of its socket because there is no socket. There is a V-shaped sacral bone, and then on either side an ilial attachment wedged against it. The whole structure, taking in the pelvic girdle, is held together anteriorly (in front), by the anterior sacroiliac ligaments, and posteriorly by ligaments holding the structure tightly in position. As you walk, the sacroiliac joint rocks along with you, serving as a sort of shock absorber. You can feel it rock. Put your fingers on the sacroiliac joints and you feel the motion. If it clicks, it is probably out of place or going out of place. You'll find nothing under your touch but some small ligaments that are the sole support of the joint. There are no supporting muscles. So when we want the sacroiliac to stay in, we advise running and walking to strengthen these ligaments.

Although there is no muscle support for the sacroiliac, muscle spasms ironically contribute to pulling and keeping it displaced. These lower lumbar and middorsal muscles, when tense, contract and pull up on the ilial or hipbone forcing it into an anterior rotation, which pulls it out of place. Thus you have a dislocation of the hip.

In measuring the ilial or pelvic bones for a displacement, both bones may be even with each other, and yet the patient feels the pressure and pain of a dislocation. For this reason we adjust or correct both joints, as both may be displaced evenly. You correct one joint first, and then discover the other must be out too because you now have a discernible pelvic tilt. So you correct the second joint, bringing the ilial bone back to position on the sacral bone. When it goes back as far as it will go, the joint locks in that position, unless it has been out so long that it has lost its original stability.

Basically, we might all be better off as far as our own backs are concerned if we crawled around on all fours, instead of standing upright, and putting the solid weight of the trunk on the delicate structure that makes up the pelvic girdle.

Anatomically, we're still in a process of change. The child-bearing female has developed a dishlike cavity in the pelvic area to carry the vital organs. But this arrangement narrows the birth canal, so that childbirth becomes difficult for a child with a large head trying to squeeze through a shrunken aperture. We have developed a strong abdominal wall, with three different layers of muscles, to support our lower organs. However, we are still susceptible to hernias because nature has not yet provided effective muscular support in the groin area to counteract the constant downward pull of gravitation.

Some anthropologists call the sacroiliac the Achilles' heel of the human back. Evolution, they point out, has not yet caught up with our upright position, with the sacroiliac sharing a double burden as not only the major locomotive joint of the body but also holding up the entire weight of the body like Atlas—without Atlas's strength or ponderosity. There seems to be a valid assumption that not long ago in prehistoric time man moved on all fours. The human embryo even today emerges as a newborn infant with a truly cantilevered or arched spine, with its vertebrae in the development stage of a four-legged creature. But as the baby develops, it loses this natural arch. The pelvis is turned upwards and shoved backwards, dropping the sacral bone between the two hipbones, instead of leaving it to form a normal tail. Since we began to stand straight, we have developed many interesting curves along the whole length of the spine. We have a reverse curve from the sacral bone up through the five vertebrae of the lumbar spine, a twelve-vertebrae arch which forms the dorsal or thoracic spine, and then the cervical spine and its seven vertebrae, which bends compensatingly the other way to help us stand straight. Living with these curves, we develop back muscles so we can bend, twist, and extend ourselves in a variety of positions. To all these natural curves, add the lateral curves of a spinal scoliosis and you've created a compound S-curve, absolutely foreign to an animal which walks on all fours. Animals are much better suited to their structure as their weight is evenly distributed horizontally, minimizing the possibility of strain. In man, there is only one cantilevered support, from the hips. With quadrupeds, we have a double spinal cantilever, supported at both ends of the body. This gives the four-legged animal the advantage of an evenly distributed suspension, without all the strain on one end.

Occasionally, a person may have a back problem, a cervical or upper dorsal curvature, independent of any sacroiliac misalignment. These conditions are usually treated by specific therapy and manipulation. For those conditions due to sacroiliac misalignment I generally don't bother working these vertebrae back in place. For once the sacroiliac is in place, eventually the whole spine will re-align itself properly, as the attending muscles gradually relax. Where there has been a scoliosis for many years, it often takes months for the spine to correct itself, even after the sacroiliac has been straightened. The period of correction varies with the individual's age and the pro-longation of the condition. The younger they are the quicker the recovery. With older people, in their seventies and beyond, even after the hip is corrected and fairly stable, it is difficult to guarantee an end to the scoliosis. The spinal resilience may be gone, the discs between the vertebrae may be harder and less pliant, the bones are softer, often porous. There may even be some change in the shape of the bone, irreversible at this stage, due to a calcium deficiency in advanced years known as osteoporo-sis or demineralization.

This calcium loss is more common in women than men. In elderly females, it expresses itself in an extreme dorsal curve, reflected in badly rounded shoulders and a loss of height. The bones have compressed in the spine, squeez-ing down ever tighter and tighter until the impressionable bones are transformed into a disfiguring hump. Some-times the bones become brittle and break spontaneously, without a fall or a blow. In such cases, it is too late for a reversal of spinal maladjustment with the corrective exer-cise. However, our preventive exercises, done regularly, would do much to slow up this aging process.

With these exercises, we shall show how one can enjoy physical well-being into the seventies and eighties, main-taining all the vital functions that make life well worth the struggle. The exercises, and the determination to do them, are an effective way to discourage chronic fatigue, headaches, colds, hardening of the arteries, stomach upset, strokes, even sexual inadequacy.

If the heart is sound, and the breath in order, you are never too old to begin, as long as you are careful not to overdo in the beginning.

You may have noticed the claim by one of the country's richest men, octogenarian oilman H. L. Hunt of Texas, that he owed his continued health and agility to making a practice out of crawling on all fours. At age eighty-three, he appeared as spry as anybody would want to be and he apparently has found a doubly-cantilevered exercise that relieves low-back tension. I have included a number of exercises in this book which I think do this job more thoroughly and effectively, but I have no argument with an exercise obviously based on the principle of reversing tension—which obviously works.

Because of gravity, the abdominal organs, intestines, liver, spleen, reproductive apparatus, all drop comfortably into the dishlike receptacle of the pelvis while we're standing, but their continued sag puts added pressure on the abdominal wall. So we try to alleviate this sag with exercises tightening the muscles in this area.

Anatomically, the spinal column is elevated above the ilial bones, the hipbones, in such a way that the total weight of the whole body is resting on two relatively small joints, the sacroiliac joints. This creates a tremendous stress in this area, making it highly vulnerable to any additional stress.

It doesn't take much for the sacroiliac to slip out. One day a young man of sixteen limped into my office. Robert was tall, well-built, intelligent, but discouraged. He had been having a lower-back problem for two years, ever since he sneezed while bending over. That's all it had taken, a sneeze at the wrong time. Now he had recurring muscle spasms so bad that he had to lie flat on his back for hours at a time for temporary relief, even after the generous use of painkillers and muscle relaxants.

He had trouble getting out of a chair, and bending over to put on his shoes. He even had difficulty getting into his trousers. He had reached a point where he was ready to give up—but he didn't have anybody to give up to.

He was in such a bad way that his mother had to help him into the office. He couldn't have made it without her support.

I gave him an over-all examination. I took the medical history, checked his blood pressure, his vital organs, the heart, kidneys, liver, lungs, and so forth. I had him strip down to shorts and socks. Then I had him take a few steps as I walked four or five feet behind him, observing his motion. I looked at the balance of fat deposits along his side to see whether one side was more wrinkled than the other and whether one side was tilted or not. The spine was slightly tilted to the right. As my eyes traveled up from the lumbar area I observed the development of a curve so pronounced that the young man was leaning in the opposite direction from which the hips and lumbar area were tilted. I also noticed that the hips were a little lower on the left side than the right.

I put my hands on the top of each hip crest and found the left hip half an inch lower than the right. This indi-

cated either a genetic short leg, a rarity, or more likely
that the left ilial bone had dropped in such a way that
the left leg seemed shorter in relation to the right. There
was considerable swelling in the lower lumbar area above
the sacrum, and this area was sensitive to the touch. I had
him lie down on his back, and checked the alignment of
his pubic bones. The left pubic bone fronting the pelvic
girdle was a full half-inch lower than the right pubic
bone. Measured together the legs were an inch apart,
giving an idea of the sacroiliac displacement. Measured
individually they were the same length, which was not
surprising.

Seeing an average of twenty-five patients a day, I
find a true short leg perhaps two or three times a year, a
minuscule percentage. Those who come in with decided
lists invariably have these lists only because of an adverse
rotation of the pelvic bone or hipbone. As soon as we
correct the pelvic rotation, the ilium—the pelvic bone—
is in absolute alignment, and the "short" leg disappears.

Robert was discouraged and disconsolate, even when
I explained that I anticipated no difficulty in giving him
relief. He had heard this story before. When Robert overextended himself originally, his hipbones had rotated anteriorly out of position. All I had to do was de-rotate this
pelvic bone, or have him do it himself. The corrective
exercise was a specific for what ailed him.

I decided to make this simple adjustment and then
show him how he could do it himself. He was in that state
where he had no confidence in his own powers. So I
placed one hand around his ankle, the other around his
knee, as in the corrective exercise, and brought his heel

above the groin at an approximate seventy-five degree angle. And then as the exercise called for, I pulled back evenly, gently. As I did so, I could feel the hipbone—the ilium—slide back into its normal position, resuming its proper apposition to the sacrum, and putting him in perfect alignment.

After I got Robert on his feet, I had him bend over a few times with his legs straight to test the stability of his sacroiliac joints. Then I put him back on the table, and lo and behold, the hipbone was out as much as before I put it in place. He would have to repeat the corrective exercise many times a day at home to establish the joint stability that he was obviously lacking at this point.

Because of Robert's prolonged problem, the muscle spasms had become part of his syndrome, and they also had to be treated. Had the displacement been corrected promptly the inflammation and swelling might have disappeared in two or three days. But new habit patterns had been set up and it might be weeks now before the muscles involved relaxed normally.

The muscles cannot stay relaxed as long as an abnormal curvature persists because the muscles then have to be heavier on one side of the spine to compensate for the extra burden that side has to bear. With this type of curvature, growing out of a prolonged sacroiliac condition, we usually find a hypertrophy (overgrowth) of muscles on one side of the lumbar spine and a diminution or atrophy of the muscles on the other side, which doesn't get as much use. So the scoliotic spine looks lopsided as you examine it and the shoulderblade may stick out an inch more on one side than the other. The ribs are a little more dominant on one side than the other, and the upper ones may be displaced.

It is not just a simple matter of your sacroiliac or your spine being out. There is a misalignment of the whole system. With a lateral curvature in the spine, your ribs don't stay even. They squeeze together on one side and expand on the other. As the pressure of this new misalignment increases, you often find difficulty and pain in the rib cage, affecting in time even the heart and lungs. You may develop an intercostal neuralgia or pain radiating around the rib cage. You may think something is wrong with your breast or your ribs, or even your heart, because of a sharp sensation of pain, heightened as you press against your ribs. Actually, in intercostal neuralgia, the nerves are irritated where the ligament supports the rib attachment to the vertebra.

The curvature causing this problem will continue to get worse if the sacroiliac joint stays out. The weakened muscles on one side become weaker. And those on the other side stronger as the demand on them increases, extending the curvature.

Because of the youthful resilience of Robert's spine, joints, ligaments, and muscles, the scoliotic nature of his spine was more readily reversible than it would be for some oldster—though it is remarkable how well people in their forties, fifties, even their sixties, respond after their sacroiliacs are straightened.

Whatever the age, ordinary common sense should be observed when back injury occurs. The individual should get off his feet as soon as possible, heeding the pain signals shooting out of this area, until he can get treatment. Almost everybody who has suffered this type of injury is usually in the process of performing a household chore or playing a game, and they usually get on with what they're doing, hoping to work out of it. By the time they finish what they're doing, they have compounded the injury.

This had obviously happened with young Robert. His back condition was considerably more painful and restrictive than originally, indicating that the muscle spasms had appreciably worsened. The problem now was that the sacroiliac, once brought to proper position, would not stay in place. I made the simple corrective adjustment as he lay on my table, angling the leg so the ilium would rotate posteriorly into place. I measured both legs again, separately and together, measured the alignment of the pubic bones, and the hipbones, and could see again that the lower back was no longer tilted. I had him stand up, and he stood as straight as anybody could. But I doubted how stable the joint would be after having been out all this time.

It is not unusual for a patient to be properly adjusted with his back in place, and then in getting off the table, again throw his sacroiliac out. The slightest stress on an unstable joint causes spasmatic muscles to pull the ilium from the sacrum to its now familiar displaced position.

I told Robert what had happened, but quickly pointed out that he had the power to stabilize his sacroiliac joint by the simple expedient of the corrective exercise. I explained the problem of sacroiliac slippage, and he seemed to understand. And then I showed him the corrective exercise, telling him that he could correct this slippage just as easily as I had.

He looked at me doubtfully.

"I have never had a failure," I told him. "Anybody can do it, and it always works."

I thought it would be easier for him to do the exercise lying down, though some, particularly the elderly, find it easier to perform sitting down or standing.

He did the exercise perfectly, clasping one ankle with his opposite hand, circling the knee on the same side with his other hand and then pulling back evenly toward the shoulder with both hands.

I told him to hold the position for a full two minutes, as his spasms were so severe that I wanted his joints to get used to their proper placement, and thus resist the abnormal muscle pull after he released his grip.

He did one leg, and then the other, and I could tell that he still didn't believe that this would do it. He had suffered too much to feel there was any easy remedy.

"In the beginning," I told him, "I want you to do this little exercise as much as twenty times a day. Do it when you get home, before dinner, after dinner, before retiring. Do it when you first get up in the morning, just before you leave for school, at the school (some empty room, if you're embarrassed), and as often as you think of it."

When he smiled uncertainly, I added, "If your injury were a few days old, two or three efforts a day would be enough to stabilize the joint. But the longer it's out, the more severe the spasms, the more fixed the error, the greater the effort to retrain the joint and the involved muscles."

Robert stood up now, testing one foot against the floor.

"Don't play games," I said, "allow yourself to heal naturally. Don't do anything in the beginning that would stretch your joints. Just move about normally, with confidence, for you now have the facility to slip your joint back whenever it goes out."

"How will I know when it's out?" Robert asked.

"At first, because of continuing soreness, you won't, so just keep doing the corrective exercise. But after a while, as the pain is relieved, you will be able to distinguish between that area feeling right and not feeling right."

"Does it make any difference," Robert asked, "which hipbone is out in doing the corrective exercise?"

"In your case both were out, and a new muscle pattern has been established," I told him. "But even if there was only one side out, I would recommend that the exercise be performed with both legs, as even with a pronounced tilt, the patient has no way of knowing which side is producing the misalignment."

The corrective exercise, I pointed out, could be preventive as well as therapeutic, strengthening the ligament attachment from the sacral bone to the ilial bone against excessive strain. There was nothing to lose by doing it. "If there is any fear that a joint might be out go ahead and do it," I said. "It can't harm you."

I had him walk around the treatment room, placing his hands on the sacroiliac joints as he was walking, so he would have an idea how his ligaments worked while he was moving.

To restore these ligaments to full operating strength I advised that, besides the corrective exercise, he should

walk three miles a day or even do some jogging. Movement is the best means of strengthening these overextended ligaments and reducing them to their original position. The walker should preferably maintain a brisk pace.
If we put stress on any part of the body, and repeat that
stress enough, without burdening the individual, nature
will strengthen that area. It may take weeks, months, but
those ligaments will get stronger—until the corrective exercise is no longer necessary, but merely precautionary.

Amazingly, a few moments after I replaced Robert's
ilial bones and had him walk around, the scoliosis that apparently existed when I first examined him completely
disappeared and the spine appeared perfectly straight
from the base of the skull to the hips. So there was no irreversible spinal scoliosis here, though a stubborn curvature would have developed in time through hypertrophy
of attendant muscles had the displacement gone uncorrected.

Sometimes, the corrected patient gets an unlooked-
for bonus—an increase in height of an inch or more. This
is no miracle—just simple skeletal mechanics. The normal
scoliosis or curvature causes a shortening in the spine,
and with the pelvic tilt you have an additional shortening.
So when you realign the pelvis and straighten the spine,
you've gained a half-inch here and a half-inch there, and
so, absolutely straight, you're an inch taller. Bob had lost
that much height, and now it was back.

Like most patients, Bob was interested in whatever
was going to improve his health, and promised to be out
walking every day.

As he was leaving the office without holding onto his
mother this time, he paused at the door and asked if he

should continue heat treatments prescribed by other therapists.

"They seem to make me feel better," he said.

"They are just about the worst thing for you," I told him. "While heat may briefly produce a sensation of comfort, it is purely transitory. Heat will only expand the ligaments, causing the unstable joint to slip out again." Instead I suggested ice packs which reduce the inflammation and contract muscles.

With heat, although there is a certain relaxation in the beginning, there is a renewal of spasm, with an increase in pain far beyond what the actual condition warrants.

Many a time, over a weekend, a patient will call me with a severe pain, saying, "I've strained my back, what should I do and when should I come in?" There's not much point describing the corrective exercise over the phone as the patient would most likely do it incorrectly. So I advise him to rest temporarily, and put icebags continuously over the area of the strain. Twenty-four to forty-eight hours later, the patient may call to say he feels fine and has no need to come into the office. Obviously there was no severe displacement of the sacroiliac, or if so, it slipped back into place once the ligaments relaxed enough to resume their normal extension.

We hear of spontaneous remissions, though it is ill-advised to count on them. Anything that thoroughly relaxes muscles or ligaments may cause a recently displaced joint to slip back—even pills that are muscle relaxers or painkillers. But they don't get at the cause, essentially a lack of tone and instability of joints and ligaments.

When a patient can't get in, I have advised aspirin, which has a relaxing effect on the body. By taking this before going to sleep, the muscles relax, and during the night, the joint may automatically ride itself back into position. The joint has a tendency to return to normal. Usually, however, the displacement is so severe that nature can't possibly do it without outside help.

I don't usually recommend rest for sacroiliac conditions. After a few days in bed, the ligaments have relaxed and lost flexibility, losing an inherent tension and resistance to motion. As these ligaments slacken from disuse, the sacrum and ilium slacken in their apposition to each other. And so, if you make an awkward turn, or pick something up without protectively bending your knees, you're apt to pull the sacroiliac out again, even two or three years after the original injury.

For the first week or so, Robert did the corrective exercise on the hour. When he returned a week later for a checkup, his lower back was in alignment, the swelling in the lumbar area considerably reduced, and the pain moderated.

After ten days or so, he was down to doing the corrective exercise two or three times a day. The sacroiliac had become stabilized as evidenced by the free and easy movement of his hipbone. He was over the hump, so to speak.

I began using ice packs for strains, sprains, and bruises years ago when I was team physician to the Los Angeles Hockey Club. We scraped ice right off the rink, and packed it on the injuries. The next day the men were out playing again despite the severity of the sprains. Since then I have never used anything but ice on any injury from a blow, fall, or strain.

In recent years team physicians in colleges and with professional football clubs have gravitated to ice therapy. One doctor in Fresno packs his football injuries in ice anywhere from twenty-four to seventy-two hours depending on the severity. The ice reduces the edema (water) in the tissues and the capillary distention, improving the flow of fresh blood to the affected area. Contrarily, apply heat to a newly sprained ankle, which hasn't even begun to swell yet, and it will blow up like a balloon. In grandma's day, before all this heat diathermy, if anybody got a bump on the head, the first thing applied was a cold silver knife or a piece of ice. Nowadays we use the ice in many ways. We can put it in a plastic bag, or take a hot-water bag or bottle half-full of water, put it in the freezer, and let it crystallize. It makes a great icebag. Or we can use these ready-made little packs they have in freezers today, a sort of picnic bag. There are plastic ones filled with gelatinous material. They hold the cold for a long period, and they get the job done.

CHAPTER III   *The Corrective Exercise*

The corrective exercise is so simple that one woman patient gave instructions over the telephone to a daughter who was not a patient—and it worked. The daughter, who lived at a distance, had moved a bed and had felt a sharp twinge in her lower back. She lay down, ironically, on the same bed to rest for a few minutes, and felt the back stiffening up. Because of the pain she was unable to get off the bed. She reached for the phone, at the adjacent night table, and called her mother. The mother, who had used the exercise to advantage, described exactly how her daughter should place one hand over the opposite ankle, and another around the knee on the same side. She told her to relax, as she either held this position for thirty seconds or pulled back evenly and gently with both hands, as too much pressure would only set up self-defeating tensions.

The daughter performed the exercise—correctly, it developed—and within a few minutes felt immediate relief. She repeated it in a few minutes, and kept repeating it through the day. In an hour or so, she was able to get out of bed without pain, her sacroiliac having slid neatly into normal apposition. She then proceeded with her housework, being sufficiently intelligent to forget about moving the bed.

Another time, a patient, who had profited through the corrective exercise, displaced the sacroiliac so severely that he couldn't even bend or move himself. He was unable to move his leg far enough to do the corrective exercise, because the pain was so excruciating. In this emergency, his wife, who happened to be a nurse, called me. It was a weekend, and I wasn't in, so she left word with my telephone message service for me to call. In the meantime, because of the continuing pain, the patient asked his wife to take his right leg, and maneuver it into the corrective position, and just hold it there for a while. It was rather awkward but she managed. She did this for him three or four times in the next half hour. And he started to feel better. He then very gingerly began to grab his own leg, and he found that the pain and discomfort were virtually gone. He was able to repeat the exercise several times.

When I called him at eleven that night, he said that he was much better, had a little ache, but was able to move about normally. He was getting ready to retire for the night and was having no trouble undressing himself. He came into the office the following morning and I examined him. The sacroiliac was in perfect position, and there was a slight spasm. I told him to continue the exercise several times a day for a week or so, and then taper off to once or twice a day. In a week the spasm and the ache were gone.

I originally called the corrective exercise the pull-back exercise because in all the years I have worked with the sacroiliac problems there has always been an accompanying anterior dislocation or displacement of the hipbone—and the corrective exercise through pulling back the leg reverses the displacement procedure by causing a posterior rotation of the ilial bone at the sacral juncture. The exercise works uniformly well because there is only one direction to go, and that's backwards. When you gently pull back the leg posteriorly and out, with a lateral emphasis you can't help but bring the displaced ilial bone into its proper relationship to the sacral bone which it is normally wedged against. Remember in pulling out and back do so slightly and gently in a totally relaxed position. The angle of 75 degrees or so at which the leg is turned into the crotch is the important thing. Just holding this angle will usually do the trick.

Usually, both hipbones are displaced in a pelvic tilt, but even when only one is involved, because of different nerve and ligament involvements, it often sends the shooting pains of sciatica down the opposite leg. It is often difficult to determine from the pain which side is in trouble because the ligaments involved may activate the pain stimuli in the opposite leg. These ligaments relate to the specific areas of pain because of tributary nerves. If the pain goes down the side of one leg, and the front, or the back, or the other leg, this is a clue to the different ligament groups and the different stresses involved.

Even if only one side or hip is displaced at first, the other may soon become affected by an uneven walking pattern, pulling at the opposite ligaments and muscles.

Not only is the person now walking unevenly, but the spine, to compensate for the tilt, automatically curves away from one side to the other. This procedure stresses on opposite-side ligaments which attach the lower spine to the ilial bone, and which affect that leg. There are also ligaments on the same side that produce symptoms in the same leg. So the pain in a particular leg may be opposite the side out of place or on the same side.

Thus it is best to do the corrective exercise on both sides, as one never knows, without expert measurement, which side is out of place. The exercise is always safe. No matter how often you do it you cannot overcorrect posteriorly by gently pulling back. You can never displace the hip posteriorly. All you can do is put it in position. And if it is already in position, you can do no harm for you are performing a helpful exercise while adding circulation and tone.

When patients' joints have been out of place on one side for twenty-four hours or so, the stress usually includes ligaments on both sides with sharp referral pains from these ligaments. As a displacement goes uncorrected, patients accumulate a familiar low-back syndrome. The spine begins making compensating changes to ease the pain and keep the person erect at the same time. The pain may be intensive, or low-grade, insistent, nagging, tolerable but a nuisance. But over a long period the average sufferer may adjust to it. In this way, they insidiously develop a definite scoliotic curvature of the spine, a pronounced S or C curve to ease the pressures on nerves and curves and satisfy the body's urge to right itself. The pain doesn't necessarily go away with this compen-

sated curvature. Sometimes it only changes the pain lo-
cale, as the curvature becomes a new spinal stress point.
But the tilting goes on, ever increasing the curvature.

In years of practice, I have found that probably ninety
percent of all stresses in the spine from the lower back
to the neck are related to a pelvic tilt from a displaced
hipbone or sacroiliac. Fortunately, these displacements
often correct themselves through a fortuitous movement,
and the persons involved may not require treatment.
They may go to bed with a bad displacement, and in the
process of twisting and turning twenty-five or thirty
times in their sleep, the displacement may correct itself,
the hipbone slipping back to its habitual sacral apposition. Within a day or two, pressure and pain disappear
and they feel fine. Other patients, unable to straighten up,
have inadvertently lifted a leg while driving or trying
to get out of their car, and then heard a click in the
lower back and felt sudden relief. In two or three days,
recent muscle spasms vanish and they talk about miracles. There are no miracles—only cures which are not un-
derstood.

In normalizing the spine, we normalize the rest of the
human body. Dr. John Mennel of Southern California,
an authority on back problems, speaks of locked vertebrae
in diagnosing spinal tensions. If a vertebra is locked in a
muscle spasm, setting up resistance to motion, the body
functions in a way to bypass that particular vertebra, and
in doing so perhaps injures itself further.

With the corrective exercise, there is an ever-avail-
able tremendous feeling of confidence. Many people with
a recurring back problem miss much of the pleasure of

life. They constantly draw back from doing things for fear of making a move that will stir up an old back injury. They don't dance, play tennis or golf, don't go swimming, or do fun chores around the house. With all this inner tension, some of it is bound to communicate itself to their bodies, making them more prone to pull a ligament or joint.

Muscle spasms normally form a protective splint for an injury. However, if the condition is prolonged, they may overprotect and produce stiffness and pain. In time, a sore, stiff muscle can be sufficiently overworked to enlarge the muscle tissue on one side by as much as a third.

Once this muscular imbalance is established, it may take months for the muscles to rebalance themselves even after the sacroiliac is corrected. However, the body is a remarkably resilient vehicle, and it will perform wonders in normalizing itself, given the chance.

I recently examined a Brentwood woman of sixty-five, who was complaining of a chronic ankle condition, marked by a painful swelling which had made it difficult for her to walk without a cane. In fact, she had the cane with her, and was eying it forlornly, as I told her to put it away, and forget it. Her condition had bothered her for eleven years, but had become more acute recently to a point where she had been limping about now for months.

I checked on her medical history, and discovered that she had fractured that same right leg forty years before. My examination of this leg showed a distorted tibial (shank) bone, presumably the result of the break that had occurred way back in 1933. The circulation in the leg appeared adequate. There was some swelling not only around the right ankle joint, but around the knee, which could have accounted for the difficulty in walking.

I next checked her hipbones. I found that she had a declination or a drop of the *left* iliac crest of about a half inch below the right hipbone. Even though the fracture was of the right leg, and the pain was in this leg, the left ilial bone had apparently been twisted out of position in relationship to the sacroiliac joint and there was a definite shortening on the left side, and the left leg appeared to be shorter than the right.

As compared to the original fracture, the ankle and knee problems were of relatively recent origin. I entertained the thought that the displacement of the sacroiliac, possibly of many years duration, could have some relationship to the bad ankle and knee. The clue came from an elevated right heel. The displacement of the left sacroiliac joint had apparently resulted in a pelvic tilt causing a ligament strain of the opposite ilium bone, irritating the nerves in the right leg in such a way as to cause the leg muscle to shorten and raise the right heel.

As I prepared to correct the left sacroiliac, I told my patient: "By re-establishing the alignment of the ilium, or hipbones, and thereby changing the weight balance on the pelvis, this painful situation may be eased, and you will become more comfortable."

I could see that she didn't understand fully what I was saying, but she was more than willing to try anything at this point.

As she lay on the treatment table, I decided I would show her even then how easy it was to correct herself. Again, she was more than willing to be shown. "Take the left leg, with its displaced sacroiliac joint," I said, "and with an overhand hold grab the left ankle with the right hand, bringing the heel of that foot as close into the pubic arch as you can. Then bring the left hand around and over the left knee, and press back gently and evenly with both hands, holding that position comfortably for about thirty seconds." I had her repeat with the opposite leg.

She did the exercise beautifully, and then repeated it a few minutes later, without any coaching from me. She was again absolutely correct in her performance, and was exceedingly careful, as I had cautioned her, not to pull back enough to work up any muscle tension that might have the boomeranging effect of pulling the joint back out of place.

I now stood her up and examined her pelvic area again. Her two ilial bones were perfectly aligned, possibly for the first time in years.

I asked her to walk across the room.

She made a little face, and reached for her shoes, which she had removed before climbing onto the table.

"I can't usually walk barefooted," said she. "I need the support of the shoe."

"Try it," I said, "you'll like it."

She made a tentative half-step forward.

"Put your foot down firmly," I said, "and see if the ankle hurts."

She made a step forward, and a curious look of surprise crossed her face.

"It doesn't hurt," she said with a smile.

"How about your knee?"

She took another step.

"That doesn't hurt either."

Though she was sixty-five, she was in good condition, aside from her leg. So I asked her if she could squat down comfortably, and then come back up again to see what the effect on the knee would be.

A little doubtfully, she got down into this fairly difficult position for an oldster.

"How does it feel?" I asked.

"All right."

"Now come up slowly and we'll see if you feel any pain or pressure."

She started to raise herself slowly.

"Do you feel anything?" I asked.

She shook her head, marveling.

"It may be the power of suggestion," she said.

"You have just undergone a change in body balance, and with both legs evenly placed on the floor, there is no pressure on either leg because there is now no short or long leg."

She complained of a certain stiffness in that right leg, and I told her it would linger a while because of the muscle spasms building up for eleven years, since she first felt the sharp pain in her ankle.

I had her walk across the room several times. "You can walk flatter-footed now," I pointed out. "Before, because of the pelvic tilt, you had to walk with your heel elevated and your toes bent."

I had to warn her, though, that this wasn't the end of it. Her sacroiliac joint would obviously be unstable because of the long time it was out, and any time she bent, twisted, or did anything to stretch the sacroiliac ligaments, there was a danger of the joint being displaced again.

"Just put it in every time it goes out," I told her, "ten, fifteen, twenty times a day to make a habit of having it in place. And eventually as the ligaments lose their stretch, the joint will stay in its normal position."

She wondered if she would ever be completely well again.

"Not *if* but *when*," I told her. "However, it may be months before the joint is completely stabilized. Ligaments are not like muscles. They are a fibrous tissue, and they are tough, but not that tough. They have been stretched a good half inch for years, and it's going to take constant correction for them to get back. But if you keep the joint in place, they'll shrink a little at a time, perhaps a sixteenth of an inch a week, until in eight or nine weeks, the ligaments have been restored to their original extension, and will hold the joint in place."

The lady walked out, painlessly, under her own power, twirling the cane as if it were a musical baton.

I followed her case with interest. She was persistent in doing the corrective exercise, making it a habit even after the ankle and knee swelling had gone down and stayed down. She put the cane away in a closet, and never brought it out again. Three months later, she was walking confidently, without the slightest trace of a limp, and with a broad smile on her face.

"I wouldn't have thought it possible," she said.

She was a walking testimonial. For she not only had corrected herself with this simple preventive and thera-peutic exercise, but she was spreading the good word to all her aching friends in her church and social circle. And they were being helped as well.

"I am afraid," she said, "that I am losing a lot of business for Dr. Thompson."

This kind of business I am happy to lose, and with luck I will lose more and more of it as time goes by. Already, the corrective exercise is costing me many old-time patients. Previously, I would treat somebody for a lower-back injury and after putting him back in place, would see him three or four times until the joint had safely stabilized. A year or two might pass, but invariably he would be back, having exerted himself in such a way as to again overextend the sacroiliac ligaments. Once loosened, the hip joint seems chronically vulnerable, and even though only a trifle out can build up pressure leading to acute discomfort and distress.

Since 1970, when I introduced the corrective exercise, my practice has been changing—for the better, I believe. It is gratifying that I can at least send patients away with a method for helping themselves when their back problem recurs. They are no longer dependent to the point where they hesitate to travel outside the radius of my office.

I do not know how many patients I have lost this way, but they are getting more plentiful daily, as witness Frank X, a tall, slim salesman, married, living a sedentary life. He first came to me in 1960, at thirty-six, with lower-back problems. Three months earlier he had an acute lumbar attack, and was taken to a hospital, put in traction, with his leg up in a sling, and given the usual heat therapy. He had severe pains down the left leg. Otherwise, his medical history was negative except for an appendectomy.

Traction hadn't helped, and he had run out of conventional therapies. I noticed a typical pelvic tilt, a listing to one side, and a scoliotic curvature in the dorsal, or midback area. As I walked him around, both sacroiliac joints showed a marked instability.

I put his sacroiliac back, and saw him a few times thereafter. I advised him to walk two or three miles a day at a brisk pace, to strengthen the sacroiliac ligaments, and advised a few stretching exercises as a preventive measure. He did these zealously for a time, but as he recovered, he gradually stopped the exercises. Four years later, he had a recurring displacement, which I again corrected, urging him to resume both the walking and the stretching exercises I advocate in this book.

He came in again in another three years. After three visits I managed to stabilize his hipbones again. He was in again a year later, and then I didn't see him until 1971. He was now forty-seven, and normally would expect more difficulty with increasing age. By this time I was using the corrective exercise. Instead of adjusting his lower back, I showed him how he could do it himself. He couldn't believe he could help himself so easily.

He asked why, if it was all that simple, I hadn't shown him the exercise before. I explained that it was so simple that I hadn't thought of it before. That seemed to satisfy him for he laughed agreeably as I showed him how to gently pull his own leg back, left hand over the right ankle, and right hand up and around the right knee, with the heel pointing almost at a right angle over the midarea of the groin. After a few false starts, he did it perfectly, and the joint slipped back into place.

He was still suffering from such severe muscle spasms that he stayed home from work for two or three days. I advised him to use this new corrective technique every hour or so for the next forty-eight hours. At the end of that time, he called to say he was greatly relieved. Two weeks later, he had cut the corrective exercise down to three or four times daily, and was holding up very well.

He gained new confidence, knowing that if he slipped out again, he could slip his hip back himself. He branched out confidently. He went in for water-skiing, which is very helpful to the general condition, including the back, when the knees are flexed to take the full weight of the body off the lower back. Ironically, the hazard was not the water-skiing, but the strain afterwards in pulling his boat out of the water. That was how he had hurt his back before, pushing his boat onto his trailer. Again he neglected to keep his knees bent—after neglecting the preventive exercises I had shown him. He came in again, I corrected him and admonished him to continue with the corrective exercise. A year has passed since I've seen him, but patient-friends tell me he is doing the corrective exercise daily and the chances are that I'll never see him again as a patient.

Like most patients, he does the exercise lying on the floor. However, it can be done effectively, sitting or standing, the important thing being that the leg be turned into the groin from the knee at the proper angle. Some patients prefer to do this exercise sitting because they are more comfortable in this position. Others prefer it standing, as a matter of inclination, though in lying down you do not have to balance yourself as you do if you are standing.

At this point, I would like to repeat the instructions for the exercise, as I feel for clarity's sake they can't be repeated too often. The exercise, lying on the back, begins with the individual grabbing one ankle with the opposite hand in an overhand hold, then using the other hand to clasp around the outside of the knee of the same leg so that the heel turns in toward and above the groin. The knee should be angled toward and slightly outside the same-side shoulder on the same side of course. Then, with the knee to heel angle at about seventy-five degrees, you simultaneously press the ankle and the knee very gently, toward the shoulder. This automatically causes a posterior angulation rotation of the hipbone, slipping the ilium back where it rightfully belongs.

Consulting the text and the illustrations in this book you can check whether you are doing the exercise properly. Though a very simple exercise it is surprising how many people after instruction do this exercise improperly. Then they come into the office, and complain that it hasn't helped. Probably the angle was not right, or they were pulling back too hard, or not using equal pressure on knee and ankle. They couldn't believe how simple it was. They had to make it complex.

Even when the exercise is done properly, as I said the sacroiliac may remain unstable for a while. I've seen corrections, on my treatment table, with the joint perfectly in place. And then, with only heavy breathing, I have seen the joint pull itself out of place. When the joint has been out a while, the tension is still so severe and the ligaments so weak that the slightest movement returns the unstable joint to a habitually improper position. As indicated previously, we may use ice to tone the muscles, relieving the tension on the ligaments, while repeating the corrective exercise at home. Again, heat, however comforting, should be avoided. I have yet to see a patient using heat who ever had a sacroiliac displacement return to its normal apposition and stay that way.

I have a few other admonitions for recently corrected sacroiliac patients. Reaching is a big no-no in the beginning until the joint is fully stabilized. Also, do not bend over with your knees straight at this stage as this may encourage the joint to slip out of place. Always flex the knees when bending over. At this critical early period, I don't advise hot baths or hot showers. Any heat tends to temporarily expand and weaken the lower-back ligaments and loosen the joint again. At this juncture I also discourage patients from reclining in soft downy chairs or lying on soft beds, as the sag encourages a sacroiliac slip out. Lastly, I don't want them extending their arms over their heads in standing position for any reason. In most of my lower-back cases, the patient was doing one of these *don'ts* when he injured himself.

Fortunately, orthodox taboos against manipulative medicine are on the wane. Physicians in internal medicine often come in for treatment, and send in friends and relatives they have been unable to help. One medical doctor, well known for her skill in Southern California, sent her sixty-five-year-old mother to see me. The daughter had heard of my work on the back through another patient of mine. She had used up all the available talent she knew of in her own particular area and was willing to try anything. The mother was at the end of her rope, emotionally. Unable to hobble in by herself, she had to be helped in by her husband and a friend. Her history was not uncommon. She had been in an automobile accident fourteen months before. Her car was backended, and she had suffered a bad whiplash. The lower back, as well as the neck and shoulder, was involved. When hit unexpectedly by two or three thousand pounds of solid metal, even though you're in a steel cage yourself, the insides are considerably shaken up. Bone, cartilage, nerves, muscles, the softer tissues, just weren't built to stand up to a steel battering ram. The medical history was familiar. The woman had had thirty treatments with shortwave diathermy on her neck, which had provided some relief. However, the lower back had not reacted to the prescribed therapy—not to diathermy, or traction for which she was hospitalized, or hot packs. I winced when she mentioned the hot packs but said nothing.

While she was in traction for ten days, she had been given pills so she could sleep, and other pills to deaden the pain. Still other pills had been prescribed as muscle relaxants, and she had also been given an orthopedic corset, buckled around her waist, to support her lower back. She still had trouble sitting down or rising. She was hypersensitive to the touch. Most of her pain was over the sacral and dorsal (midback) area. After more than a year of this, she was understandably depressed.

I didn't have to search very far to find the difficulty. The scoliotic changes in her spine were plainly visible. There was a severe lumbar (lower back) curvature and a

lesser distortion in the midback. Standing her up, I saw
the telltale pelvic asymmetry. The iliac crest (top of the
hipbone) was rotated anteriorly out of place, presumably
from the jar of the collision. After correcting the displacement, I put her through the usual walking motions, which
revealed that the sacroiliac joint was unstable and would
slip in or out without much prompting. The moment she
got up or sat down, the joint displaced itself again, and
the strain on her sacroiliac ligaments would bring back
a spasm of acute pain. She also complained of pain in the
cervical spine, at the neck.

All I corrected was the sacroiliac. And this is all I had
the patient correct. I explained to her that I was rearrang-
ing the pelvic asymmetry, allowing the spine to adjust
itself to a normal position, so that the normal curvature of
the spine—lumbar, dorsal, and cervical—could re-establish
itself.

She was a special problem because of her age and the
prolonged period of sacroiliac slippage. Her holding ligaments were not as resilient as a twelve-year-old girl's, or
a young man's of twenty-five. But she wasn't bad for her
years, and she had a strong inner urge to get well and become a useful citizen again. Because of the deterioration
of muscle function, I did not think it wise in the beginning
to allow her to treat herself without supervision. So I had
her do the corrective exercise at home, meanwhile having
her come into the office for additional treatment. For three
weeks, I applied corrective procedures, loosening up her
muscle spasms and aligning the joint, which was still
highly unstable. She began to get relief not only from

lower-back pain but in the upper back as well, and we didn't even touch the upper spine.

As the pelvic bones stay aligned for any length of time, the irritation and pain correspondingly subside. After a month or so, she was feeling well enough so that she didn't have to come back any more.

"I feel confident now," she said, "that with the corrective exercise I can take care of myself."

She said this without bravado, but with a smile reflecting the wonderful transformation she had undergone with no more pain to worry about. Where she was depressed before, in the space of a few weeks she had become a stimulated, happy, gay person, ready and eager to pick up the threads of a productive life.

As a precaution, we decided she would come in once a month for a while. On her next visit, which was the last time I saw her, she was in perfect alignment, both in her pelvic area, and in her serene view of life.

Sometimes the results from correcting the sacroiliac are so instantaneous and sweeping that even I am surprised. One day at a friend's home, I met an attractive television actress, who had been complaining about a chronic sinus condition. Her name was Jeanne Avery.

The friend looked at me impishly.

"Try your corrective exercise on *that*," he said.

"Her sacroiliac is probably out of place," I replied. "Nearly everyone's is at some time or other."

Miss Avery was a good sport, if slightly incredulous.

"Do you mean you might help my sinus by straightening out my hip?"

"It's happened," I told her.

She cheerfully stood up for inspection. Even through clothing, I could discern that one side stuck out more prominently than the other. There was a deeper indentation at waist-level on the left side than on the right. One shoulder was higher than the other and her head tilted to one side. Even without looking at the spine the body posture clearly indicated a misalignment of the sacroiliac with a spinal curvature.

She regarded me anxiously.

"What's wrong?" she asked.

"Nothing that can't be easily corrected. You are just a little on the bias. There is an uneven distribution at the hips, waist, shoulders, and of the curves at the neck. Everything is distorted."

Miss Avery's eyes bugged. "You mean I have all that?"

Our host seemed to enjoy the impromptu consultation.

"Would you like to go straight?" he asked the actress.

"I certainly don't want to be the way I am, now that I know how I am." She gave me a puzzled glance. "But what does all this have to do with my sinus?"

"We shall see," I said, entering into the spirit of the occasion. "Meanwhile, if you will lie down on the couch, I will check out your pubic bones."

The host seemed to find this amusing.

"It is the simplest way," I said, "of determining pelvic asymmetry."

Sure enough, as I suspected, Jeanne's right pubic bone was three quarters of an inch lower than the left. She obviously had a sacroiliac displacement of long duration, and her spine had compensated with a definite lateral curvature, which could affect not only her posture but her breathing and general health.

I decided to show her the corrective exercise.

We began with the right leg, and I instructed her to hold her right ankle with the left hand, and clasp the right knee with her right hand. "Just lie comfortably, and either hold the leg at this angle or pull back easily and evenly, allowing the muscles to relax so that the joint will slip back into place by itself." She held this position for about thirty seconds or so. The ankle was gently pulled toward the midsection and the knee meanwhile slowly moved back and out without exerting any pressure. At this exaggerated angle in the pullback or hold position the ilial bone turns posteriorly and slides into normal position.

Jeanne did the exercise perfectly. She kept her left hand over the right ankle, and her right back and around the right knee. And her position was just right, her right knee angled back outside the line of her right shoulder, the heel above her groin. She held the position for forty seconds. I checked her out again. Ilial and pubic bones were absolutely symmetrical. There was no need to do the other side.

She sat up and began testing her hips.

"I feel freer than I did," she said. She kept testing. A one-time Yoga student, she tried slipping into the Lotus position, crossing each foot over the opposite thigh. She gave an exclamation of satisfaction. "Previously in the Lotus position, one leg would never go down, but now it does."

There was no longer a constriction in the hip or lower back.

"How often should I do this exercise?" she asked.

"You can do it as often as you like, ten times, a hundred times or one time, depending on how you feel."

She looked up curiously.

"But how does this affect the rest of me?"

"A sacroiliac displacement often brings about somatic changes. The ligaments of this joint under stress may produce a somatic nerve impulse which affects the viscera—the heart, liver, lungs, and primarily the intestines—which in turn cause a change in peristalsis and a change in the cells that produce secretions in the intestines."

She looked at me doubtfully.

"Over the years," I went on, "I have observed a definite connection between a corrected sacroiliac and improved gastrointestinal function. Within a half hour, or even minutes, some patients have reported relief from chronic gas spasms. The sphincter muscles, affected by the sacroiliac adjustment, have relaxed sufficiently to release the gas blocked by spasms throughout the intestinal tract."

Jeanne was still testing. Now, pointing to a flower in the room, she spoke in astonishment. "Just a few minutes ago, before I lay down, I couldn't smell that rose. And then the corrective exercise began to work on me, I began breathing easier and suddenly I felt my sinuses drain. I could hardly believe it. I had been gasping for air. Now I find myself taking huge gulps of air. I haven't been able to do that for years."

My friend eyed her curiously. "She does appear to have a fresh radiance about her, her eyes are glowing, and she seems vitalized. But it might only be imagination—hers or mine."

I was gratified by the transformation. "This is another of those somatic changes I was talking about," I said. "The sacroiliac adjustment, relaxing the spine, eased tension in the rib cage, relaxing the lungs once again in a free and easy symmetrical pattern."

Jeanne nodded. "That's been my fight, to get those lungs loosened up so that I could breathe properly, and get rid of allergies that have bothered me so long."

"As you get enough air," I told her, "you'll have more energy and more resistance to overcome your allergies."

Our host was still skeptical. "I just don't see how a sacroiliac adjustment can influence the breathing apparatus."

"It all goes together," I told him. "It's all one body, and every cell and nerve affects every other cell or nerve, drastically with a sudden change in body pressures. With the sacroiliac out of joint, the rib cage is cramped on one side and expanded on the other. This causes the body to exert itself to co-ordinate the rib motion to the automatic rhythm of breathing, often resulting from this extra effort in shortness of breath and premature fatigue.

"So many people with a chronic sacroiliac problem complain that they are tired all the time. They just can't get going. After the sacroiliac joint is stabilized, they happily report they have all the energy in the world because they are breathing freely again. For the first time in a long time their breathing is co-ordinated with diaphragm, lungs, and rib motion. Previously, the diaphragm at the bottom of the rib cage had been somewhat suppressed as a result of rib restrictions. There is a feeling of being locked in at both ends, diaphragm and lungs. Now once you straighten the spine, relieving the oppressive curvature in the spine, the rib cage, lungs, and the diaphragm function normally and you can breathe deeply without effort."

CHAPTER IV

Straightening Out Children

The baby was three months old, cute as could be, except for the ominous fact that she was thin and undernourished and couldn't hold down her food. Even the mildest formula—and mother's own milk—refused to stay down. The worried mother consulted the baby doctor, and he thought that a change of formula might help. It didn't. The child continued to throw up as one diagnosis after another proved fruitless.

As both parents were patients of mine, they finally decided to bring the baby in to me for a fresh opinion. After checking the child out routinely, I looked at her lower back and hips. In my practice, vomiting is common among patients with displaced sacroiliacs. Lo and behold, as my eyes wandered over the tiny torso, I could plainly see a pelvic tilt, and a scoliosis, lateral curvature of the spine. The displacement was slight, but enough to result in discomfort and distress for so small a child.

Various pressures build up inside, as the nervous system reacts to distortions of the spinal column. Often the individual feels nauseous. An infant can hardly describe its own symptoms, but in this case there was enough wrong with the child's back to explain her indisposition.

I laid her on the treatment table and quickly put her hip in place. She was a model patient, eying me curiously with her wondering blue eyes as I moved her tiny legs in the corrective exercise. As we didn't speak the same language, I could hardly tell her how to do the exercises. But it was a simple task to instruct her mother, so that she could adjust the sacroiliac in the event it slipped out again, a procedure I would not ordinarily recommend except for a helpless infant child.

Minutes later, for the first time in two weeks, the vomiting ceased, and there has been no recurrence since.

Sacroiliac slippage is not unusual among babies. Their hips may be displaced in a difficult delivery, their bones being so pliable at this stage, or they may take a bad roll in the crib and wrench themselves.

When a child has a sacroiliac or scoliosis problem, it is vitally important that it be caught promptly. Otherwise, the curvature of the spine will become inherent in the growing pattern, and little can be done later. The problem may start at age two or three, and if not caught by age four or five, it may already have developed a fixed scoliosis pattern. By eight it may be too late, as it may have become an established part of the child's formation and development. Usually, the problem isn't noticed until the child goes to school, and gym teachers notice a droop in a shoulder, and a lateral distortion in the upper spine. As a rule, the child has not complained of a back problem because the tendency to pain and stress is not as great, since the curvature has blended into an adolescent growth pattern where the tissues are softer and more flexible, as nature intended them to be for their own expansion.

When the displacement first occurs, either through a fall or strain, the child may show some distress. But as he adapts rather readily, and the pain quickly passes with his soft tissues accommodating a new alignment—or mis-alignment—the condition is allowed to continue without attention from the family. Eventually, there will be some slightly noticeable changes or spinal curvatures which the parent feels that the child will outgrow, until finally the child is examined one day, usually for something else, and the therapist says, "Oh, we have a bad scoliosis here and we are facing a possibility of surgical intervention."

And he is probably right, for not only has the spinal curve become part of the child's natural growth, but the rib cage usually shows an asymmetry that verges on de-formity. What could have been easily remedied, with a few simple spinal adjustments, and the regular use of the corrective exercise, can only be corrected now with drastic methods—with braces and lifts and possible sur-gical interference.

Somebody once said an ounce of prevention is worth a pound of cure—and never was an expression more ap-plicable to a situation. Every parent should take especial notice of their growing child's posture, particularly be-tween the ages of two and eight, before spinal changes become part of the *normal* growth pattern. The parent should keep a watchful eye for any particular deformity—a change in the curve of the spine when the child is stand-ing, or one hip being a little more prominently placed than the other, or as when a dress or trousers hangs from one hip a little higher or lower than the other. The difference may be slight, only a quarter of an inch, but a quarter of an inch is quite a bit of sacroiliac displacement in a child and can gradually produce an even greater change in the curvature of the growing spine. The child should be examined periodically to make sure his pelvic bones are growing evenly. If they are even as he is growing, his spine will be straight in adulthood. He will have no back problem, as a rule, until he becomes an adult and displaces his sacroiliac in doing something his muscles and ligaments weren't prepared to do.

If the displacement isn't caught, between the ages eight to eleven, resulting scoliotic changes usually develop with opposing shortening and lengthening of the tissues alongside the sacroiliac joint and the spine so that the curvature is now an ingrown process. It cannot be altered through simple manipulation. However, adults, eighteen or over, whose bones have already formed straight and true, may pick up a scoliosis which continues for ten years. But, if the ilial bones are then evened up, the scoliosis as a rule will eventually correct itself.

There is no way of telling the proportion of children with premature curvatures. But we do know there is a large number of scoliotic children going through corrective surgery between the ages of twelve and sixteen. Even worse off, of course, are the adults with virtual deformities which are an outgrowth of a childhood scoliosis that went unnoticed. Their sacroiliac joint is invariably out and we can relieve the stresses in the lower back due to this displacement. But the scoliosis is so fixed by childhood neglect that the spinal bones have grown in a curved pattern with a narrowing at one side of the bone that just can't be reversed with exercise or manipulation.

In surgery, doctors usually fuse the bones in as normal an alignment as will be tolerated, using bone from elsewhere in the body to accomplish this fusion. Of course, the spine will not become fully straight and there will be a loss of flexibility. So even this drastic treatment reminds us of the importance of preventive procedures, which are purely academic unless the problem is first noticed and treated.

Since the problem often develops after a child suffers a bad fall, it would be wise to check the child's lower back area for a pelvic tilt immediately after the tumble and for a week or two thereafter. Sometimes the sacroiliac slips back naturally as the child makes some propitious natural movement, but often it doesn't, and these become the cases we are concerned about. It is very easy for a playing child to hurt himself in such a way as to throw his hip out. I recall one case where a six-month-old baby fell out of a crib—a not uncommon occurrence—landing in a sitting position. Both sacroiliac joints (as we later discovered) were displaced with a great deal of pain. The mother didn't know what was wrong with the child. The little girl kept crying for no noticeable reason. The mother related it somehow to the fall, and brought the child to me. The child's hips were quite tender, and she let out a scream at my touch. My measurements indicated that both sacroiliac joints were severely displaced or dislocated, and the joint showed an unusual laxness. Her little backside had received quite a jolt. I corrected the hips, and then wrapped a special binder around the child's lower back to support the loose sacroiliac ligaments. I had not yet worked out the corrective exercise, but even so, because of the unusual instability of the joint, some extra help was needed to retain the corrected position until muscles and ligaments properly healed. As the child wasn't walking yet, it didn't have the benefit of regular motion to strengthen these ligaments.

In three or four weeks, nature had done its healing work, and the binder was removed. By catching the displacement promptly, a potentially harmful scoliosis had been averted, and our six-month-old patient was as good as new.

I would suggest that therapists check a child's spine and sacroiliac as a matter of routine. They look at the child's eyes and ears, the feet, chest, teeth and heart, but ignore one of the most vulnerable areas. For falling down is almost an occupational hazard in childhood, and nasty falls can displace sacroiliac joints so severely they may never correct themselves. As it is, about the only children with bad spines that I see are children of patients who know from their own experience how prevalent and disturbing a lower-back problem can be. Promptness in treating children with displaced ilial bones cannot be overdone. With children, it generally takes a year or two for the spinal curvature, resulting from the sacroiliac displacement, to actually alter the density of the vertebrae and the pads of softer cartilage or discs between the vertebrae. After two years or so, with small children, the scoliotic change is usually irreversible without surgery, which at best is not totally effective. In these cases, X rays show a very definite shortening of the vertebrae on the inside of the spinal curve. Also, when the spine has been scoliotic for a long time at this impressionable period, one group of ligaments may become shorter than the other, because of the constant lateral pull. Even worse, there is now little chance of their ever being lengthened because the improper growth pattern has become inherent in the bone structure. Time after time, I have seen seventeen- and eighteen-year-olds whose scoliosis has been ingrained in their skeletal system, and I must regretfully explain that they have come in several years too late. The curvature, along with a cramped rib cage and drooping shoulder, has become a part of their nature, and it is difficult to reverse nature.

The less time the child has had its displacement, and resulting scoliosis, the easier it is to correct. The parents of a five-year-old girl noticed there was something just not right about her spine. The spine just didn't seem to have a normal curve. One pelvic bone seemed a little higher, and a new dress didn't hang right, bulking more on one shoulder than the other. It was a marginal situation. The child hadn't been complaining, as the ligaments and tendons at this age often are so soft and pliant that they yield painlessly to stress after the spasm of the original injury has passed. And this may leave in a day or two at this age.

The parents decided not to chance their daughter's growing up crooked. If the examination was negative, what was to be lost? At least, they would not have that to worry about. So they came in with the little girl. With one glance, I could tell her sacroiliac was out on one side. The displacement was a recent one. But even had it been two or three years old at that stage, the child was still sufficiently unformed so that her bones and cartilage could have been stabilized and retrained. But had she been over eight years old, and the condition an old one, the improper growth pattern might have been so advanced that the spinal curve could not have been fully reversed.

As it was, I corrected the sacroiliac, and walked her around my examining room five or six times to observe the motion of her hips. Within five minutes of the correction, her pelvis evened up, easing the pull on her spine. The spine straightened in front of my very eyes. Eighty percent of the scoliosis had disappeared before she left the office, and in another week or so the spine was completely straight.

Brisk walking helps in the reconditioning process, once the sacroiliac is replaced, because the hip motion encourages the spine's natural tendency to correct itself. The easy rocking motion often helps the joints and ligaments to ride back into normal apposition.

I showed my five-year-old patient the corrective exercise. Children usually can manage it themselves at the age of four. I also showed the parents how to do it, so they could make sure the child did it correctly. In a few days, the child was back to normal.

I emphatically urge parents to check their children's spines carefully, as the condition is so easy to correct in sacroiliac cases when caught right away. They may show the child the corrective exercise even before seeking professional help. Within ten minutes after being adjusted, the child who was nauseated or in lower-back pain may walk around freely saying, "I feel fine now."

It can't possibly hurt the child to do the corrective exercise. The exercises are beneficial even if the sacroiliac isn't out. It's a good stretching routine, increasing circulation and flexibility, if nothing more.

Both children—and adults—could profitably do the corrective exercise every day, after the Yoga-type program we recommend or after walking or jogging. The chances of developing severe back problems would be vastly minimized, and the individual might forestall visceral and other somatic problems that arise from a sacroiliac condition.

The somatic symptoms from a displaced sacroiliac are almost diagnostic in nature. The first thing I do with a child with a bellyache is to check the sacroiliac. Irritation in the sacroiliac ligaments apparently affects neighboring nerve roots in such a way that a disturbed sacral plexus has an adverse effect on the intestinal function. This of course applies to adults as well.

Examples of this somatic relationship are commonplace. A young mother telephoned one day because her four-year-old boy was clutching his stomach and complaining about a tummyache.

"How is his back?" I asked.

"It's his stomach," she said, apparently thinking I hadn't heard her correctly.

I asked her to bring him in, knowing that she would not likely detect a pelvic tilt, nor be able to do anything constructive about it if she did.

When he came in that afternoon, he was still holding

onto his stomach and crying miserably. I checked him for possible appendicitis and other abdominal complaints. They appeared to be negative. The mother's concern seemed to deepen as I turned the boy over and began examining his back. He had a decided pelvic tilt, a moderate curvature of the spine, and the left leg was about a half an inch shorter than the right one. I stretched him out on the treatment table, still wailing, and put his sacroiliac back. It slid back easily, perhaps too easily—it was that loose.

He stood up rubbing his eyes, as I explained the visceral somatic syndrome to his mother. She listened politely.

We had talked about five minutes when I turned to the boy, who had stopped weeping, and asked, "How's your bellyache?"

He smiled. "All gone."

The boy's abdomen had been distended by gas, apparently reacting to spasms formed by the intestinal pressures touched off by the sacroiliac displacement. Often, within a few minutes after the joint straightens out, the patient may hear a gurgling in his stomach and have a sensation of relief as the gas pains begin to break up.

Some somatic changes from this displacement are more subtle in nature. The same boy was suffering from a severe rectal itch, and the mother thought it caused by pinworms, as there had been a mild epidemic in the neighborhood. Since she couldn't bring the boy in that day, I suggested she check him for pinworms first. I told her to apply a piece of Scotch tape over the boy's anus just before he went to sleep that night, and check it in the morning for pinworms. Pinworms usually come out during the night to provoke this itching. She found no pinworms. So I advised she bring the boy in for a checkup. She made it that afternoon. I looked the boy over, and saw that his lower back was out. I slipped his sacroiliac back in and the next day the itching stopped. But the joint was unstable, as it had apparently been out for some time, presumably from a fall. And so it took two additional treatments, with the corrective exercise applied at home with the mother's help, before the joint became sufficiently stabilized to maintain its original position.

In such cases, by no means unusual, the rectum is obviously affected by a nerve impulse touched off by a spasm from the sacroiliac joint. Had the mother gone to a doctor not familiar with the wide impact of sacroiliac displacement, the boy might still be taking medicine for worms he never had.

It is hardly ever too early to begin a helpful all-around exercise program, with the corrective exercise part of the preventive therapy. When a child reaches school age, five and a half or six, he is capable of doing our Yoga-type exercises for increased flexibility and stamina, proper breathing, improved co-ordination, and concentration. Concentration is particularly important when a child is just beginning to develop a pattern of study. Children need to be shown the importance of a sturdy body as the repository of a sound mind. It is never too early to put emphasis on health rather than sickness, on exercise and gyms rather than doctors and hospitals. Preventive medicine is the best medicine. We should stress with children the value of encouraging good health rather than waiting around helplessly to get sick and then doing something— if it isn't too late or too costly. When we prepare for a voyage on a ship, we put in provisions and instruments and all the things necessary for a safe journey. Why shouldn't we prepare our bodies with similar foresight for a safe voyage through life by giving our bodies the proper nutrients, the proper exercise, and the proper spinal resources so essential to our motor and somatic function? By improving circulation, body tone, respiration, and endurance, we automatically increase the body's resistance to disease. And this applies particularly to children, who have not lived enough to build up the immunity to infection that the average adult has. They have not had as much exposure, and may be more susceptible to drastic temperature changes, bacterial invasion, and environmental pollution. Nowadays, it takes a strong stomach to overcome the incessant barrage of food poisons, bad water, and polluted air, notably smog. If we are to endure life as it is today, with its foul atmosphere affecting our physical activities, we must compensate accordingly to maintain increased stamina and resistance. With better health and endurance, heart and lungs become stronger, more adaptable, we breathe easier and better, receiving more of the oxygen we need to cope with an incompatible environment.

As the tissues get tougher in relationship to the environment, they may eventually overcome even the abnormal stresses the environment puts on the human cells. We build up resistance gradually. If we want to lift one hundred pounds, we start perhaps by lifting the twenty-five pounds that we can manage without excessive strain. By gradually increasing the weight pound by pound over a period of time, we eventually reach the point where we can safely lift the hundred pounds that would have been too heavy for us in the beginning. We have made the body adapt itself to changing conditions by relating it intelligently to increased stress. This adaptability under carefully measured stress is as true of the heart and lungs as it is of the skeletal muscles. If we increase the stress factor by gradually increasing the body's ability to handle that stress, we muster a greater ability to handle a given load at a given time, usually far in excess of our first aim.

Because of greater vulnerability, it is even more important to get children on a sound exercise pattern than it is adults. The exercises we outline, particularly those relating to improved breathing, may make it possible for the growing child to withstand environmental stress that would ordinarily induce disease malfunction. As the child —or adult—begins to do these exercises, his breathing will noticeably improve, giving him an advantage in dealing with the smog and in fending off emphysema. Anything that benefits lung expansion helps it resist infections localizing there. Youngsters who could hold their breath but ten or fifteen seconds are soon holding for a minute or more, indicating a strong beneficial improvement in expansiveness of lung tissue. Where smog is a problem, many experts have argued that the individual shouldn't breathe deeply. In Los Angeles, during smog alerts, people are cautioned not to overexert. However, there is a significant difference between exercising and overexerting. In our exercises, expanding the lung power, we minimize the possibilities of overexertion, and prepare the body for the stress smog puts on the entire system, not only the breathing apparatus. By expanding the lung tissue you allow the lungs to work to their fullest extent, increasing their elasticity to their ultimate utility. By increasing lung capacity, the individual gets more oxygen in a restricted situation, such as in smog. Anything that increases the total capacity of the lungs obviously increases its oxygen intake, and lessens the possibility of an oxygen deficiency, permitting the body to adjust more easily to environmental or muscular stress. Mountaineers living in the thin air of the high Andes, have compensated over the generations by developing an unusual lung capacity to handle the greater amount of air needed to offset a reduced oxygen mix. Their rib cages frequently become larger than average to accommodate the necessity for increased expansion. In time, because of persisting smog, our own lungs may adjust to handle atmospheric impurities and lowered oxygen content. But we haven't accomplished this evolutionary change as yet. In exercising their lung capacity to their fullest, with the help of deep breathing techniques described in our exercises, children will expand rib cages, ventilate sinuses and nasal passages, and increase their endurance while aerating their lungs with the precious oxygen they can't live without. We may be taking in a little more smog in deep-breathing, but it is a small price for the oxygen desperately needed in a polluted world. In an emphysema condition aggravated by smog and cigarettes, the lungs doubly need oxygen to function properly, as irritated tissue, unable to expand normally, drastically reduces the lungs' breathing capacity.

All this is further complicated by a scoliosis, resulting from a sacroiliac displacement, which restricts the normal rhythmical movement of the rib cage in breathing. It is bad enough to have the smog, emphysema, and consequently a restricted lung capacity, without the added burden of scoliosis' cramped ribs and the somatic changes that affect the viscera, including lungs and heart.

All in all, this is perhaps the most important chapter in this book, because it bears on the happiness and futures of those just starting out in life. Every child can be helped before it is too late. And every child has the right to grow up straight. It is not only a matter of physical but of psychological health as well, the two eventually merging anyway.

Many children, particularly girls, as they reach puberty become increasingly conscious about their appearance. One such young lady was brought to me by her parents, not because she had a crooked spine, alas, but because she was in constant pain because of it. Another therapist had fitted her with a lift in her shoe to correct a curvature which became socially noticeable when she was ready to wear her first spring formal to her first high school dance. The dress, instead of showing off her slim youthful figure, instead accentuated her bad posture, the unevenness of her hips, the dropped shoulder, the pronounced lateral curve of her spine.

I don't approve of lifts normally, but in this case the evil was doubly compounded by the lift having been placed in the wrong shoe, apparently from an error in reading the X ray. Had the lift been placed in the left rather than the right shoe, it would have at least evened up the pelvic tilt, without of course getting at the seat of the problem.

The first thing I did was toss the lift in my waste basket. I then corrected her sacroiliac. Fortunately, it was a rather recent displacement. The pain disappeared almost immediately, but the joint was unstable. So I recommended a couple of more visits, where I could judge her progress, with the corrective exercise meanwhile being done at home. She did the exercises faithfully, and when last I saw her, a month after her initial visit, the disfiguring curvature had completely disappeared.

She was all smiles when I suggested she would be the belle of the ball at her next high school formal. And so, thinking of her and many others, like her, I hope every parent in America will remember:

"Your child has the right to grow up with a straight spine."

CHAPTER V

Always on Monday

Monday is my busiest day. Monday is the day of the weekend athlete. Mondays are emergency cases, patients racked with pain, unable to stand straight, because they have done something to their backs. They were just fooling around the boat, or gardening, bowling, playing touch football with the kids. And then, suddenly, or perhaps gradually, they find their back is acting up.

"What happened?" they ask. "I've done this thing a thousand times before."

And they have, but not with the same muscles, ligaments, and tendons. They were doing something their bodies were no longer used to doing, with tissues that had lost their elasticity. They actually weren't the same tissues they had when they were doing all these things with effortless ease.

If they had exercised properly, regardless of advancing years, it would not have happened. They put excess stress on the body and the tissues gave. Mostly, they suffered strained ligaments in the lower back, or displaced sacroiliacs. These were not true accidents, though tissues atrophied from disuse often make people susceptible to accidents. They were the normal casualties of a normal American weekend. All week the weekender gets in shape bending over his desk, taking a cocktail or two at lunch, later sprawling at home in front of the television watching football or baseball or a late movie, "exercising" with a can of beer in his hand. He has reached an age, the late thirties or early forties, where he no longer finds time for a gym, and yet his muscles are still as big and strong as ever. They have just lost their resilience. The ligaments don't stretch as they used to, and the muscles tense with toxic accumulations that a diminished arterial circulation can no longer easily carry off. The heart, like other major muscles under unaccustomed strain, becomes easily fatigued and contributes to an over-all stress which is a perfect medium for injuries.

Weekend mishaps take many shapes. Skiers beat a path to my door. Like bowlers, they may be young, middle-aged, old. This demanding sport puts stress on the most expert and the best-conditioned. With a fall or twist, practically the trademark of this exhilarating sport, skiers often displace the sacroiliac and a painfully constricted back results. Younger skiers, prone to disregard injury, plunge bravely down hill and dale, aggravating an unstable sacroiliac joint and encouraging a scoliosis of the spine.

I sympathize with youngsters who have traveled hundreds of miles with expensive equipment to some beautiful ski lodge, and understand why they will do everything, short of skiing on one leg, to keep the weekend going. Now with the corrective exercise they finally have the ideal tool to manage this, without fear of extending their initial injury. It's just a matter of getting it to them.

One young lady, an expert skier, had taken a tumble, and pulled her sacroiliac. She came into my office hardly able to walk, much less ski. Her total incapacity had saved her from hurting herself further.

After I showed her the exercise, she felt prompt relief. That next weekend she was back skiing. She now noticed, as people often do with bad backs, how many other skiers had back complaints. She passed on the exercise to them, and before that weekend of fun was over skiers lined up in queues at her hotel room for treatment. They were all young weekend athletes who had put a strain on ligaments and muscles after some inactivity.

Fortunately, they were treated while their joints were stable enough to immediately respond. Often, the joint has been displaced so long that stretched ligaments lose elasticity, and the joint won't stay in place. Prompt replacement of the joint is important along with some recognition of one's own suitability for the task at hand, whatever it may be.

The weekend gardener is hardly in the precarious class of a broken-field runner when he gathers up his spade and begins putting in the petunias. Yet he may suffer more damage than a Joe Namath or a Fran Tarkenton before his weekend is over. He operates on hands and knees, a demanding position to which his de-toned ligaments and muscles are long unaccustomed. He stays in this crouch for a while, not feeling any particular discomfort at the moment. Then he tries to scramble to his feet, and realizes with a start that it isn't as easy getting up as it was getting down. He strains a little to get to his feet, and then may feel a slight crimp in the lower back. It is nothing, he tells himself, but he has to exert himself to straighten out. He is now a low-back casualty, with a displaced sacroiliac.

It could all have been so easily avoided. Had he done our rejuvenation exercises daily, even five times a week, he could have squatted all day and his tissues would have been resilient enough to handle this awkward position. Had he known about the corrective exercise, after he injured himself, all he had to do was lie down a minute or so and pull each leg back in the prescribed angle, and the sacroiliac would have slipped back into place.

There is a popular misconception of what good physical condition implies. People in shape for one activity are not necessarily conditioned for movements employing a different set of muscles and ligaments. Frank X., a contractor of forty, a husky individual who was always doing heavy lifting, carpentry work, or plumbing, gloried in his toughness. Super-confident of his powers, he was as strenuously active on weekends as during the week, dune-buggying on wild stretches of Pacific beach, water-skiing with the kids, even giving volley ball and touch football that old college try.

One weekend he took a bad bounce on the dune buggy at a Pacific beach, and his sacroiliac promptly slipped out. Another time he pushed against his boat when he should have pulled. The last time he was in, I showed him the corrective exercise and stressed the value of Yoga-type conditioning exercises. "In this routine," I told him, "we consider the body's total relationship to stress."

Even though these exercises do not impose a great deal of strain overall, we are stretching, bending and twisting daily, giving the involved joints and ligaments a tensile strength that permits weekend stress. Our preventive routine emphasizes flexibility, as constant flexing of neck, shoulder, spine, hips, knees and ankles makes these areas more resilient than ever.

This contractor accepted the exercise routine, including the corrective exercise, and I haven't seen him for a year now. Previously he came in every three months or so with a banged-up shoulder or displaced hip. A certain flexibility of mind, which made him open to suggestion despite an overweening pride in his physical prowess, helped him achieve a corresponding flexibility of body.

Sometimes a back is so bad that the individual can't even play on weekends. Jack T., a tall beanpole of a young man, was quite fragile, at six feet five and 150 pounds. His family brought him in because his spine was developing an abnormal curve. The right shoulder had dropped three inches lower than the left shoulder. He looked like he was hauling a hundred-weight of coal on one side. He was so off-center and so much in pain that he wasn't able to play tennis, golf, or even bowl with comfort. A musician by trade, a cellist, he had worked part-time as a truck driver, and in moving heavy loads off the truck his slender frame had adjusted to the strain. His right side, assuming the dropped shoulder, had reacted to the excessive demand. His chest was bulging with muscles on this side, as was the scapula or right wingbone. He was a rather one-sided young man. Working full-time as a musician after his trucking experience, he found that sitting a full evening left his lower back stiff and uncomfortable. Besides that, he lacked his old co-ordination, and didn't play as well.

My examination showed a severe sacroiliac displacement of about an inch. Heavy lifting over an eight-month period had carried the discrepancy to the upper spinal area. Looking at his distorted rib cage, I wondered how he could draw a deep breath, and he did find it difficult to breathe normally, resulting in constant fatigue not only from lack of oxygen but from the required effort of constantly gulping air.

I corrected the sacroiliac, which was highly unstable, improving his upper lateral curvature or scoliosis, and showed him the corrective exercise. I then asked him to take a deep breath. The surprise on his face was gratifying. He was bringing the air down to the bottom of his lungs for the first time in a long while. With the rib cage cramped on one side by his scoliosis and expanded on the other, there had been a definite resistance to normal expansion and contraction of the ribs during breathing. In normal inhalation, the diaphragm goes down, and the rib cage expands to effect increased expansion of the lung tissue. When the air is exhaled, the diaphragm comes up and the rib cage contracts. The young man had not only been starved for oxygen because of the restricted motion of his rib cage, but was mentally depressed by his inability to get a satisfying breath of air.

Although the restriction wasn't totally removed in one treatment his breathing was immediately responsive in proportion to the new freedom of motion in his rib cage. With his rapid scoliotic response to the sacroiliac alignment, his posture was fifty percent improved as well.

It would take weeks to stabilize the sacroiliac and fully bring his breathing to normal, but I knew he would be back for additional treatment. For the first time in months, he felt light and airy enough to try his hand at golf or tennis. We had another weekend athlete to contend with, but at least he knew about the corrective exercise.

The ladies, too, have their weekend problems. As mentioned, gardening can be dangerous if the gardener isn't in shape for it. And the ladies like their gardening.

As the keeper of the home, the female spends many more hours around the house than her spouse. She is cleaning, mopping, washing, familiar tasks which do not usually provoke problems. But every once in a while she may want to shove around some heavy piece of furniture. Wanting to surprise hubby when he gets home, she may ambitiously move about a bulky chair or sofa, or rearrange a carpet or rug.

Her muscles may be strong enough for the task, but the joints and ligaments frequently aren't up to the stress. Too busy to exercise regularly, she does very little walking and will jump into the car to drive a block to the grocery store. Consequently, there is no reserve strength in the sacroiliac ligaments, and the affected joint will give before the furniture does. She may come into the office all bent over, moaning about getting old before her time. One look at her spine tells the story. Besides the telltale list to one side, she usually has a spinal curve resembling a big S.

In the midst of her cleaning chores, one hardy lady in

her thirties decided to move the family piano. As she tugged and heaved, she felt a slight kink in her back, but not until the next day did the back strain manifest itself. She told herself bravely, "It's going to get better." Two or three days later it was only worse. For as the joint stays out of place, muscle spasms become continuous, and the scoliotic spinal curvature increases with the pain.

She phoned for an appointment. One look indicated the sacroiliac. I slipped it back in position, showed her the corrective exercise, and advised ice packs to reduce the inflammation. If she was careful, in five or six weeks the displaced joint would be stable again and the pain disappear.

The healing process is one of nature's wonders. Every fiber of a ligament or a tendon has an adjacent nerve fiber and blood vessel or capillary. When you hurt yourself these tiny tissue fibers become irritated, and the nerve fiber picks up this signal. The body's response is one of pain.

Blood rushes to the affected area to begin the healing process. Where the injury is severe, the pain increases as the circulation is blocked by the edemous swelling around tissues which are inflamed. Ice is valuable in treatment of inflammation, reducing the edema and permitting the healing blood to resume its normal flow to the tiniest nerve and ligament fibers, encouraging that proliferation of fibrous tissue which knits bone, cartilage, and flesh together.

Whenever stress is put on tissue not adjusted to such stress by previous conditioning, that tissue can be grievously hurt, and this applies to the heart—the most vital muscle of all.

If an individual has not exercised regularly and put an *unaccustomed* strain on the heart, his heart may over-react to new demands with unfortunate results. As other unconditioned muscles, the heart is laden with fatty tissue, and fat anywhere in the body constitutes a vulnerable area. As muscle shrinks with disuse, fat fills in the gaps. In such a situation, normal for the middle-aged or the younger in sedentary occupations, too much caution cannot be observed. If a man sits at his desk for two or three years, his only exercise walking to the car or bus, and then is called upon to run half a block—yes, half a block—in that little distance he can put enough strain on his heart to cause serious damage. In an emergency the heart picks up its beat to supply oxygen for the strenuous exertion the body is not used to. The overworked heart just can't handle the extra volume of blood and a coronary may result.

We shouldn't immobilize ourselves for fear of damaging our hearts, but instead mobilize our physical resources —blood, muscle, bones, nerves—to keep our hearts strong for the challenges of life. Just as fat forms in the heart tissue from inactivity, it disappears with the right exercise program. The human system takes fat from all parts of the body, for energy to run the human machine. Fatty heart tissue serves no useful purpose. Fat-formed deposits interfere with muscle motion and vascular circulation, reducing the heart's ability to contract as it should.

Prepare your body every day for what it has to do. Give the blood a chance to circulate, and keep the blood vessels healthy and elastic, so they adequately nourish the heart and lungs. When the heart isn't contracting properly, pushing the blood to the rest of the body, the general health suffers. But as a staunch muscle, the average heart can take a lot of abuse. However, too many people as they get older suddenly stop the competitive sports that have developed their heart muscle instead of prudently tapering off to a less vigorous routine. As the heart's work slackens, and calories increase, useless fatty tissue adds to the aging heart's burden. Exercise is a preventive as well as a corrective measure.

After a coronary recovery, many doctors recommend regular exercise, jogging, swimming, what the patient should have done before his attack to maintain a constant exertion trimming the fatty tissue and providing an adequate blood supply to the heart.

I strongly recommend the group of stretching and breathing exercises in this book, beginning easily with only the mildest of strains. Do only a few exercises at first, gradually stepping up repetitions and adding exercises from this series.

The routine should be done regularly. The only exercises that help are the ones you do, not those you talk about. If you put any muscle, including your heart, under slight daily strain, if only for five or ten minutes at first, the more likely you are to keep your heart healthfully responding in conditions of stress. Our bodies are habit-trained; as long as they function in their habit pattern we have nothing to be concerned about.

Just observe a few common-sense rules. Before you break into a run, ask yourself when you last ran and what distance. Our rejuvenation exercises will condition you for running, but not if the stress of running is vastly greater than the stress of the conditioning exercises. As an example, I had been trying to get one of my middle-aged patients to do some exercise. He hadn't done any in years, and he was getting a pot belly. I reminded him that he couldn't have any fat outside without also having it inside. Have you ever picked up a chicken, already cut open, and noticed all the fat inside? Or have you noticed meat with marbleized fat between muscle and tissue? We humans have a similar tendency. My paunchy patient was in his early forties, and quite strong of limb, but he hadn't done regular physical exercise in years. And then one day, having forgotten something at the market, he dashed across the street to pick it up. He never made it. He was just stepping off the curb when a sharp pain stabbed his chest, and he collapsed in the street. He ended up in the hospital with a coronary, and was there for weeks. Recovered, he is now exercising moderately and in time his heart will be stronger than before.

As you observe tissue's uniform response to injury, you realize how much alike human beings are. Essentially, men, women and children, black, white and brown, are of the same physical essence, and their bodies respond similarly to stress. It is the minds that vary, and the spirit, that indefinable quality a doctor senses in patients, which is often his supreme ally in effecting a quick recovery. After treating thousands of patients for every conceivable ill, I have decided that as man thinks so largely does he function. Right-thinking is the priceless ingredient, and it affects the weekend athlete as it does every patient who comes through my door. The patient's will to get well has made many a doctor look good. While tissue has its similarities, the challenges, obstacles, and conditions vary with one's station in life. The lawyer, the engineer, the streetcleaner, the housewife, all are subject to different stresses.

Housewives are probably the most overworked and underrated of people. And they are more prone to weekend disasters because as a rule they don't keep even as fit as men do—and they do more sporadic chores, including gardening. Mabel F., a forty-year-old housewife, had a chronic back problem for two years, which made her a setup for a sudden disaster. One day I got an emergency call from a relative. Could I come to Mabel's home in Los Angeles right away? She was in such pain that she couldn't leave her bed. The pain was girdling her waist and shooting down her leg. She was in agony, and panicky because she couldn't move herself.

She had spent Sunday in the garden, pruning the weeds and undergrowth, planting some new flowerbeds. She had straightened out suddenly, and then collapsed. They had to carry her into the house, and roll her onto the bed.

I got to her place that evening and found the family had not exaggerated. Mabel couldn't even go to the bathroom. They had brought a bedpan to her room, and even this presented difficulties.

Examining Mabel, I saw that she had done herself considerable damage. The sacroiliac was out about an inch and a half, a maximum displacement, and painfully protective muscle spasms had formed around the injury. I put her hipbone back into place, but it was obvious to me that with the slightest movement it would slip out again. Fortunately, I was now using the corrective exercise, and I showed her how to do it, telling her that she could use it as often as she liked, every ten or fifteen minutes in fact.

With most of the pain now eased by my adjustment, she was ready to try anything, particularly since she could at least amuse herself in bed with this exercise. It worked out very well. In three or four days, doing the exercise faithfully, she was able to leave her bed and come into the office. The stress, swelling, and pain from the strained ligaments were still present. Even though I had corrected the position of the ilium, the hipbones, the affected sacroiliac ligaments would be sore for another two or three weeks. They had received a traumatic shock, and would recover in their own time. I used ice to reduce the inflammation, and suggested she make an icebag out of a hot-water bottle, and apply it continuously at home. The reduction of the swelling made it easier for her to get around and reduced the period of discomfort. Meanwhile, she went ahead with the corrective exercise, and in two or three weeks she was able to move about without any pain at all. Feeling back to normal, she thought she was ready for the garden again. I advised her to begin the preventive exercises outlined toward the end of this book. However, she did these for only a few days, and then discontinued them, laying herself open for another attack. For some reason, women do not take to regular exercise routines as cheerfully as men. I suspect the male is prodded by the romantic ideal of a strong, virile body, and works to stay younger longer to satisfy his picture of himself as a great lover.

While weekend athletes may be any age, the casualties seem to favor the forties and fifties. People in their twenties are often still active physically, and those in their thirties are just growing out of youthful activities and so are not quite so stiff as those in the older brackets. In the thirties, many still bowl, dance, date, still participate in group sports, are still in gyms. Their jobs are more active. Not quite up in the business echelon they haven't reached a point where they can sit around and give orders. They still are running and fetching. After thirty-five or thirty-six, the average person begins to find himself slipping physically. And to compound this loss, he cuts down sharply on his physical activities. More than advancing years slow him down. His kids are a little older and he's not out with them any more, hiking, fishing, sailing, as they've reached an age where they've either discovered girls or prefer to be with boys their own age. At forty, he begins to fall a victim to the national psychology. He tells himself youth has passed him by. He starts to think of himself as older, except for those impulsive weekends when he tries his hand at painting or fixing things around the house or boat. Or he may even decide that he will resurrect the glories of his youth and take a hand in some pickup game with the kids. At forty, there is usually a marked decline in physical strength, and any strenuous activity is a strain, unless the individual has been exercising regularly.

If he does the exercise routine every day, he can do what he wants to do weekends. I can testify to that myself. I have always been hesitant about advocating any course I don't practice myself. I can truthfully say, nearing sixty, that I can exercise freely on weekends because I do my preventive exercises every day. I seldom have a cold or indisposition of any sort, and every weekend I am on my boat, painting, sanding, working around the engine, washing down the sides and deck, pulling and hauling. After a day of this and a refreshing shower, I feel great. However, if it weren't for the stretch exercises keeping ligaments and muscles supple and sinewy there is no doubt in my mind that I would have become a casualty long before this. I am no superman, merely a physician who has learned the wisdom—in this instance —of practicing what he preaches.

There are as many ways a person can hurt himself as there are human activities including sex. The ancient Romans, who ruled with a heavy hand for centuries, were of the opinion that the sex act could be performed as an exercise. They were dedicated to physical fitness and mental soundness, and they stressed in their day of glory the quest for bodily improvement. By their standards, we are a generation of weaklings, and the sexual act, rather than strengthening modern man, often results in physical debilitation, even to inducing a bad back. Many patients rather sheepishly report strained backs during intercourse. I assure them there is nothing to be ashamed about. In the actual contact and motion of sex, it is possible to suffer a strain in such a way that a sacroiliac joint can be displaced with one twist of the torso. After two or three days, if the sacroiliac does not rock back of its own volition, the individual becomes increasingly uncomfortable, and is well-advised to subordinate his embarrassment and get help.

Sex, normally, is not hazardous, and it wouldn't do for loving couples to restrict their love-making because they aren't up to the Romans. Copulation is a perfectly normal human function intended by nature to be as pleasant as it is. It is rarely injurious to the back, except through overly exuberant exchange of caresses, with perhaps more enthusiasm than any physical act really warrants. Many patients have described in clinical detail the gyrations that led to their aching backs. And listening, I have only wondered that they did so little damage. But they seem to have found it interesting.

Curiously, I find more sexual casualties resulting from clandestine romances than from the ranks of properly married couples. The reasons are not as esoteric as they might first seem. Where the sex act is furtive and illicit, particularly if the people involved are not with their marriage partners, there is a certain underlying tension stemming from guilt or anxiety. And this tension communicating to the body interferes with the rhythm and co-ordination so essential to relaxed movement. With sex, as any exercise, tightened ligaments and muscles may eaily lead to bodily overextensions causing a slippage in the sacroiliac joint, situated as it is in a highly vulnerable area.

Although weekend sports, without a daily exercise preparation, are a precarious route to pleasure, there are certain athletic pursuits, such as hiking and bicycling, that can be helpful, provided they are done regularly every weekend. Both activities, begun moderately, build up

THE
CORRECTIVE
EXERCISE

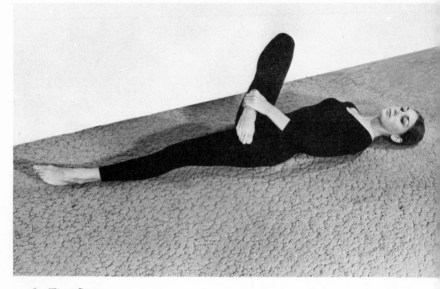

1. First Stage

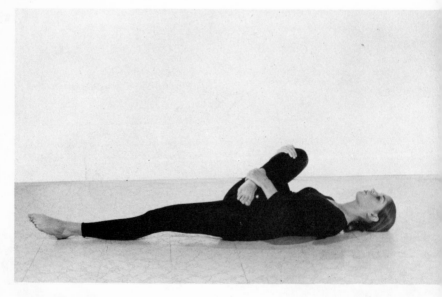

2. Second Stage

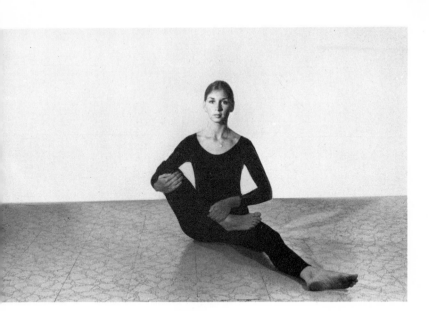

3. Sitting Posture

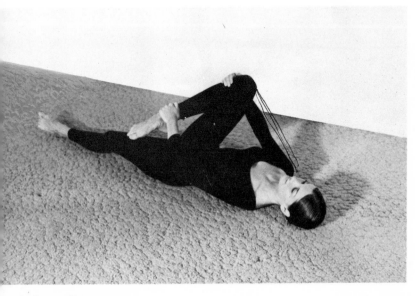

4. Lying Down

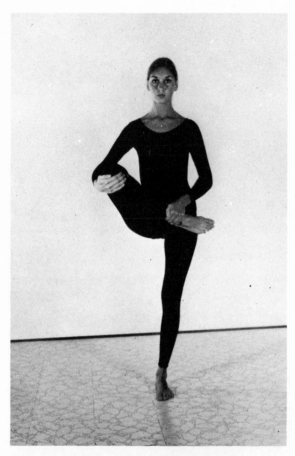

5. Standing

OUR REJUVENATION EXERCISES

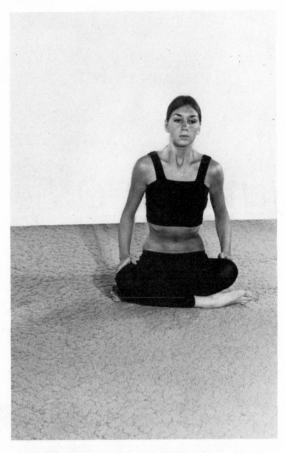

6. Deep Breathing—Stomach Contracted

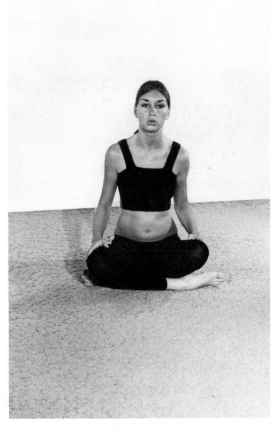

7. Deep Breathing—Stomach Out

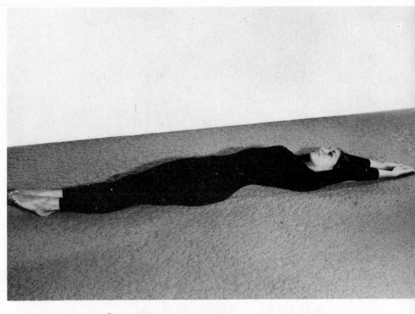

8. Spine Stretch

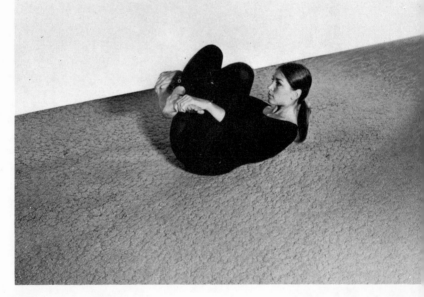

9. Rock 'N Roll

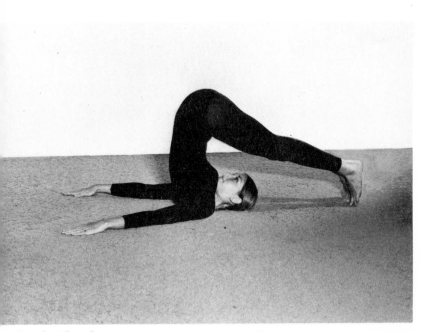

10. The Plough

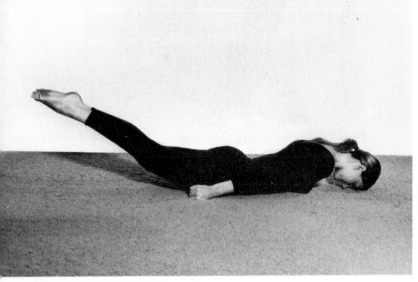

11. The Locust

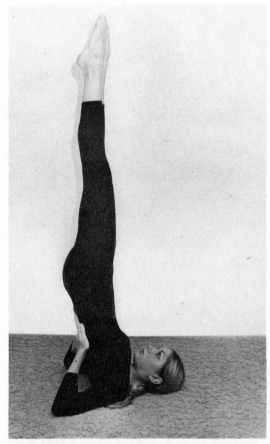

12. The Shoulder Stand

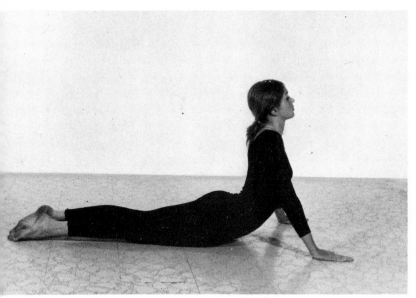

13. The Cobra

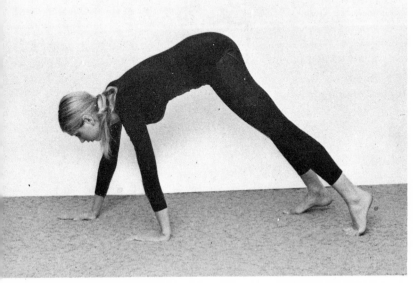

14. All Fours

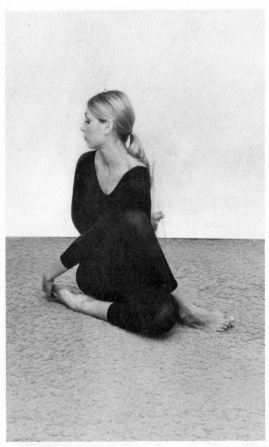

15. The Body Twist

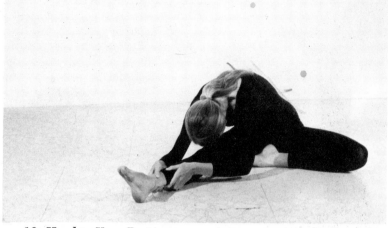

16. Head-to-Knee Posture

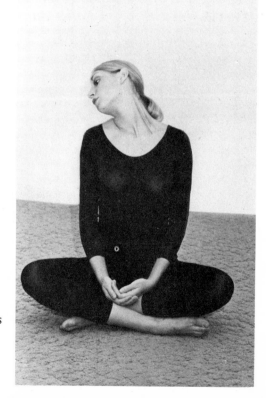

17. Neck Rolls

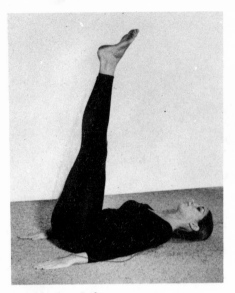

18. Leg Lift

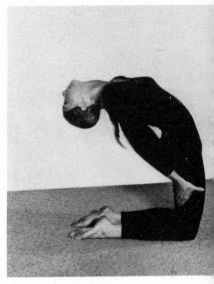

19. Knee-Back Extension

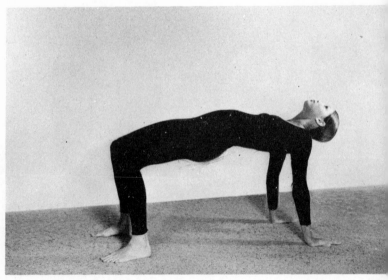

20. The Table

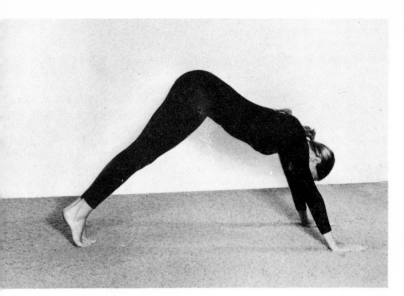

21. The Cat

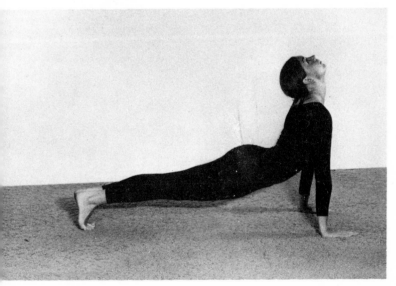

22. The Cat

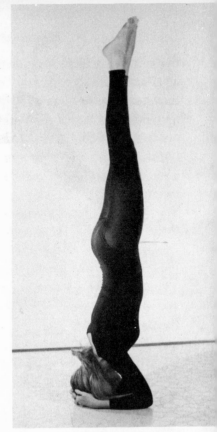

23. The Headstand

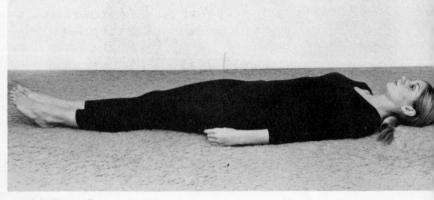

24. Peace Posture

the critical sacroiliac ligaments. However, some middle-aged cyclists have thrown out their sacroiliacs because they had done nothing for years to keep their bodies toned up before ambitiously embarking on the open road.

Every weekend athlete should know his own limitations. One patient, a lawyer, in his midforties, had become intrigued, as he drove along the Pacific coastline, by a caravan of keen-eyed cyclists pedaling single file. The cyclists included not only the young but many as old or older than himself. But he failed to note the flat stomachs and steely legs. The oldsters had earned the right, through disciplined conditioning, to ride with the young. Our lawyer got himself an English racing bicycle and shot out of his garage one Sunday, headed for the Pacific Ocean. A half hour later, straining with might and main to reach the crest of a hill, he felt a twinge in his back. It got worse as he kept pedaling, until he had to slide off the bike and walk alongside it. And this was also a painful process.

He limped into my office the next morning. Both ilial joints were displaced and he had a considerable amount of spasm in the hip area. After putting him back in place, I showed him the corrective exercise and Yoga-type exercises I find so rejuvenating. "Work on these a while," I advised, "before you take the bike out of your neighborhood."

In bicycling over a distance, the sacroiliac is particularly vulnerable. The legs and hips are in constant motion, but there is little low-back support because of the cyclist's practice of leaning forward over the handlebars. In this position it is particularly easy to overextend muscles and ligaments. However, bicycling, done properly, is great exercise for the legs and the arms, the wind and heart, particularly with bikes with hand-type brakes that work on the arm muscles. Once the individual is in shape for bicycling, he can stay in shape by bicycling once or twice a week, especially if he is doing our conditioning exercises during the week.

Golfers are among my favorite patients. They usually report on Monday after a frustrating weekend in which they took out their frustrations on a little white ball. I see tennis players, touch football and volleyball addicts, skiers, skaters, and sundry other weekend athletes, but the golfer is my prize. Although tennis is a more furious game, I get three times as many golfers as tennis players. Many of these are excellent players, and in good condition. The nature of the game has a lot to do with their problem. Any golfer has a tendency to occasionally misjudge his swing, usually straightening one leg too soon and taking his weight off the leg itself. By locking the knee, instead of bending it a trifle, the golfer puts all his weight on the sacroiliac, as the thigh is no longer involved in the swing. All the force of his swing is now related to the upper buttocks and the lower back. And these are the areas where unaccustomed stress may shift the ilial bone, forcing it anteriorly from the sacrum.

The more serious-minded the golfer, the more likely he is to throw himself out. Any time anybody is tensed up, emotionally or physically, he is vulnerable to a sacroiliac displacement. The mind quickly transmits its tension to the body. Muscles tense and tighten, the leg stiffens, and the swing instead of being an easy synchronized motion, awkwardly thrusts the entire weight of the body on the sacroiliac at the very time the golfer is extending the lower-back ligaments involved in his swing. People usually don't relax as much with golf as with other sports. Bringing their competitive spirit from the office or factory, they're usually more concerned with achieving a low round than with the exercise, the fresh air, and the sun. One fifty-year-old business executive I know was in better shape than most weekend golfers. He loved to play golf and he managed to play two or three times a week. Yet, he was a regular patient, with a constant, recurring sacroiliac displacement. In view of his excellent condition, and regularity of his play, I couldn't understand why he was repeatedly injuring himself. I would correct him, he would go out and play a few rounds, and back he was again. I sat him down and questioned him about his game. From what he told me, I realized that he was so inherently tense and tight that he couldn't really play a relaxed game. He would play eighteen holes, perfectly relaxed, with everything going well. And then he would start on a second eighteen. Perhaps a little tired, he'd bogey the first or second hole, drive into the rough a couple of times, and start to get annoyed with himself. His annoyance would communicate to his swing, which also tightened up. And the next thing he knew, he took another swing and his lower back was bothering him.

I showed him five or six of our conditioning exercises to stretch and relax his ligaments and muscles, inuring them to sudden strain. He started doing them, and his "golfer's back" seemed to disappear. And then one day he was back again. He had been doing the exercises every day, feeling better, and then he had decided he was well enough now to discontinue them. I put back his sacroiliac and told him that if he really wanted to stay out of my office, he should make a daily habit of the exercises. I gave him the Yoga-type twist, the Plough, the Head-to-Knee, the Cobra, and the back-arching Table. I told him to do each one, slowly and gradually, and not to extend himself. In time, he could absorb the complete routine. He apparently learned his lesson, and has not been back recently. I could have told him not to get upset and to concentrate on relaxing, but I have found it easier to change people's bodies than their minds.

Like the golfer, the tennis player has a specialized problem. Surprisingly enough, it isn't tennis elbow, a painful tendinitis from excessive strain, but the simple fact he isn't in proper playing condition for fast tennis. The game itself does little to prepare the lower back for sudden bending and extending. If the player were walking five miles a day while playing tennis, his sacroiliac joints would be properly resilient. But as a rule, the weekend player grabs a racket after a long layoff and bustles out on a court, ready to challenge a Billie Jean King or Pancho Gonzales. As in golf, the trouble-trigger is the swing. In swinging, the player who keeps his knees flexed, and his legs springy, is not liable to hurt himself. But the moment he stiffens his legs and bends or twists, stiff-kneed to return a serve or smash, he invites a painful wrench in the lower back. I get more tennis players with bad hips than bad elbows. Tendinitis in the elbow is a long time building up whereas the hip can come out at one fell stroke.

With tension, there is not only a tendency for the player to hurt himself, but to foul up his game. This holds true in virtually all competitive sports. In professional baseball or football we often hear the taunt, "He's choking up." Not a very considerate observation, it may even accelerate the choking-up process. The weekend athlete should constantly remind himself that he is playing for fun not blood. He should be out for exercise and fresh air, in a mood of light contention. And only with this attitude should he approach the game, and every move while playing it.

Unless you are free and easy, and can throw off your problems, you are better off sitting down and brooding somewhere alone rather than hurting yourself at some game under the pretense of getting away from it all.

Total relaxation is one of the best defenses we have against sprain or strain. Remember the story of the drunk who fell down a flight of stairs, then picked himself up unhurt (asking who had pushed him) because he was totally relaxed from the numbing effect of the booze. I don't recommend this for anybody, athletically inclined or otherwise, but it does point up the value of relaxed muscles and ligaments. The average person in the act of falling downstairs would immediately tense up, and so break a few bones or tear a few ligaments. So relax completely in playing a game or in doing anything that requires a physical commitment. You will last longer.

CHAPTER VI   *The Sacroiliac Blues*

Not long ago, the parents of a twelve-year-old schoolgirl brought her to me in sheer desperation. She had developed a severe side pain, which seemed to bother her most when she exercised in class. She complained to her teacher, and the teacher, thinking it might be appendicitis, sent her home, advising the parents to consult a doctor. The parents took her to one doctor after another. The physicians could find nothing wrong. After three or four doctors had examined her, the school doctor had a look and concluded as the others had that her problem was imaginary.

"There is nothing here physically," he decided. "She needs a psychiatrist."

By this time the girl was indeed troubled. She had a constant stabbing pain, and she was being told there was nothing bodily wrong with her. It was enough to depress anyone, even if she hadn't already been depressed by the mysterious pain that kept her from participating normally with her schoolmates. After a while, she couldn't concentrate on her schoolwork, and this began to build a whole new syndrome of ineffectiveness and uncertainty. The thought of the future began to terrify her. Would she be able to go to college like other girls, work and marry, and have children one day herself? It all seemed so uncertain and so forbidding, and here she was only twelve.

There was no question at this time that she was disturbed emotionally. But what twelve-year-old, or adult, wouldn't have been in the circumstances?

All Georgie could think of at school after a while was the pain in her side. She became alternately defensive and panicky about it. "I do have something wrong with my side," she kept insisting. "It does hurt."

The girl's parents were almost as troubled as she. The idea that she might have something mentally wrong with her horrified them. They were beginning to wonder about themselves, for where else would a girl that young acquire a mental problem. Reluctantly, they set about checking out the available psychiatrists they could afford. It looked as if they were all in for a long, rough haul. They still hadn't decided what to do when a close friend, who was a long-time patient of mine, suggested they bring the girl in to me.

She was a pretty little thing, and she didn't appear much different from other girls her age who were my patients. As a physical-oriented doctor, I looked to find something physically wrong that would justify that constant pain in the side—and I found it.

It took only a minute or so to discover her pelvis was tilted, and the sacroiliac stretched out of joint. I put her hip in place, and the side pain, a referral from the sacroiliac, disappeared. She returned to school and that ended the problem. She never did get to a psychiatrist.

The girl's case was not unusual.

Repeatedly, people with low-back problems are told that they are emotional cases, merely because the problem is not viewed in its proper physical perspective, and their very real pain is glibly attributed to "nerves."

Of course, in time, any unresolved back problem may very well become an emotional problem. The ancient Yogis were far ahead of their time when they postulated mind and body as one—the Sanskrit term Yoga itself, meaning yoke or union, exemplifies how closely the two elements are interrelated.

Often stress brings on an emotional problem which becomes a back problem and then reverts to an emotional problem again. Patients develop a tremendous sense of insecurity and fear when they complain of a painful back and the practitioner cannot find anything wrong in that area. After an examination that proves negative the family doctor may advise X rays. And the X rays may not show anything that they can read or evaluate in terms of their own experience. Even if there were a sacroiliac slip, it would not be revealed by looking at the sacroiliac joint on an X ray. The pictures would only show pelvic asymmetry, one hip higher or lower than the other. But this would mean nothing to the average technician or doctor, because he isn't looking for it and likely wouldn't know what it portended if he did see it. So the orthodox therapist may tell the patient, as so often happens, that he can find nothing wrong. "I don't understand where the pain is coming from. We'll just have to wait and see if it goes away."

After a while, finding no relief, the patient goes to another doctor. This doctor looks him over and also finds nothing. "It must be a muscular indisposition, perhaps arthritis."

He is probably right about the arthritis, since many people in their thirties, forties and fifties do have some arthritis. Arthritis is a combination of body stresses. As we get older, these stresses, reacting chemically within the body, often build small bony spurs, calcium deposits, on the edges of the spinal vertebrae. Early arthritic changes are usually minor and present no symptoms, and the patient may or may not react to treatment. However, the patient with a slipped sacroiliac is complaining about something that can be readily treated and corrected, and treatment for arthritis isn't going to help his sacroiliac or his sciatica.

Having run the gamut of medical doctors, the patient may begin to believe what friends and relatives are telling him—that it is all in his head. He may even make an appointment with a psychiatrist—back sufferers are doing this all the time. The psychiatrist has no concern with the back. As far as he's concerned, the patient has an emotional problem, or he wouldn't be there. By now the patient is so thoroughly confused that he does have an emotional problem, aggravated by the likelihood that he can no longer work, or even get to the office, without hobbling or twisting about in pain. As psychiatric treatments continue without relieving his back, he becomes more and more depressed. And the psychiatrist by now is sure of his diagnosis. He's really got a full-fledged case of melancholia on his hands. But invariably when he sees that psychiatry isn't helping, and the drain on his pocketbook is excessive, this type of low-back patient leaves the psychiatrist and begins to doctor himself with drugs. He's taking drugs not only for his back, but by now for his nerves. He's a mess, he knows it, but he doesn't know what to do about it. He's desperate. At this point, luckily, he meets up with somebody who's been through the same thing, but has come out of it when his sacroiliac was put back in place, and the stress on the ligaments—and the attending nerves—was automatically relieved. I have seen it happen time after time with people. The depression quickly leaves, as confidence comes back. They don't have as much fatigue, their bodies become relaxed and stronger. The pain vanishes.

Many patients have taken to drink over their aching backs. But perhaps they might have found another reason for drinking if their back hadn't bothered them. Low backache over the years, with its incessant pain and restrictions, gives a sense of inadequacy which often leaves one vulnerable to drink or drugs. I make no moral judgments. My only function is to help if I can, not sermonize.

A lady alcoholic in her forties came to me with a painful back problem she had had most of her life. Curiously, it coincided with her drinking problem. She was not suicidal but close to it. She was married, but the marriage was in turmoil because of her drinking. She was always contrite, guilt-ridden, remorseful—and in pain. She just had a feeling of not being able to cope. She would drag one leg after another, howl with pain when she bent to pick something up. She had seen more doctors than a board of medical examiners. She had no sense of purpose, no hope—only the bottle, and this in turn was only making her feel worse.

She was recommended to me by another patient. My first impression was that she had not come in expecting help, but only to oblige a friend, whose persuasive insistence had finally overcome her own reluctance. It was the way she ran her life, choosing the least line of resistance.

I gave her a thorough examination, and then checked over her back. The sacroiliac was out. I would have been surprised if it hadn't been, for with the occasional exception of spinal tumors, I have seldom had a case of lower backache where the sacroiliac wasn't out.

I put her back in place, and showed her the corrective exercise.

She seemed relieved that I had found something physically wrong with her. Still, she was incredulous that so simple an exercise, done readily at home, could correct her back problem.

"It won't if you don't do it," I told her.

She had complained of being chronically tired, and fatigue and depression go hand in hand. When the sacroiliac is out, the trunk is no longer in a relaxed, restful position, and even in repose, lying or sitting, there is a constant sense of muscular tightness, along with pain, which is fatiguing in itself. Also, with chronic fatigue the body chemistry changes, and the individual gets the toxic blues. The curvature of the spine, interfering with the proper apposition of the ribs, also reduces the breathing capacity of the lungs through adverse pressures, and there is an

oxygen inadequacy, not only fatiguing, but rather un-
nerving to people who panic over catching their breath.

I made no attempt to explain all this to my lady alcoholic. In its complexity, it might have driven her back to
the bottle. Instead, I told her that her pain problem and
any attending problems, were attributable to a displaced
lower back. I had her do the corrective exercise until she
appeared to have mastered it, and I sent her home full
of hope.

As I wanted to monitor her progress, I had her come
back once a week. At the end of the third week, she had
undergone a complete personality change. For the first
time since she was a girl she had developed a confidence
in being able to do things. She cut down on her drinking,
and supplanted "the sauce," as she put it, with our little
exercise. She was a new woman. And, as I told her, if
the corrective exercise did nothing else, it would enable
her, if she relapsed, to enjoy her drinking more.

When the sacroiliac is out for any time, the nerve plexes
in critical areas are directly affected by somatic changes.
Many patients become nauseous, and vomit without apparent reason. Some are affected in other disagreeable
ways. Possibly because of bladder reaction, many women
with a displaced sacroiliac have a constant, embarrassing
need to urinate. Perhaps because of the difference in the
urogenital tract, the male bladder is not affected as much
as the woman's. But then women ordinarily have more
bladder problems than men do. Traveling anywhere in a
car with men and women, you discover that it is the
ladies who are constantly popping into the roadside rest-
rooms. They seem to want to stop every few miles. But

with their sacroiliacs in shape, the mileage between stops is vastly increased.

While a bladder problem may be upsetting, it certainly doesn't frazzle the mind and spirit in itself. I have found that the tension and emotional disturbance level of the average patient coming in to see me for the first time varies with the length of time his condition has persisted and the number of doctors he has already seen. These long-term sufferers are not only in pain and somewhat incapacitated but troubled, insecure, fearful, confused—all adding up to a man-size depression. Most of them have been told that sooner or later if their conditions persist, they will require surgery, and myograms—a myogram being an electrical test of the impulse of a nerve stimulus to a given muscle. Almost without exception, these patients are at a point where they have tried every approach and have reached the end of their rope. They are desperate people, afraid they will never get better. "You are the last," they tell me. "If you can't help me, I quit."

Some have felt good one day, getting by twenty-four hours without pain or stricture, and then, suddenly, without their doing anything, the pain and discomfort has come back. What they don't realize is that because of their long ilial history, their sacroiliac is so unstable that one moment it may be in place, and the next slip out by itself.

Some have had surgery and that hasn't helped and that makes them doubly desperate. One young lady had a disc removed in a fusion, pieces of connecting bone transplanted from another part of her body to immobilize the offending vertebrae. She had hoped this was the end of her problem. She was relieved for a short time, and then the pain and spasms returned. When I looked at her, her sacroiliac was still displaced. I corrected the displacement, showed her the corrective exercise, and suggested she do it at least ten times a day, until her joint was stabilized. Removal of the disc had removed the pain focus at that particular point, and it turned up elsewhere. The operation had not done any good. As mentioned elsewhere, except when there is motor loss and paralysis, I don't see any benefit in fusion or disc removal at any time. The corrective exercise, simple as it is, helps almost any functional back problem. And it helped hers. In a few weeks, the sacroiliac had stabilized, her spine had straightened, and she was as cheerful as a June bride. The darkness had dropped out of her life and she could hardly believe it. It had been so easy. Nevertheless, she had to work at it. It takes at least three days for the muscle spasms to relax comfortably. Until the sacroiliac is retrained through constant repetition of the corrective exercise to stay in place for a corresponding period, the pain continues, with the possibility that a wrong move may pull the hipbone out again. So she had to keep putting the joints in place until the joint stabilized sufficiently to give the needed muscle relaxation. The muscles were sufficiently relaxed by then not to pull on the sacroiliac ligaments and start the vicious cycle all over again.

If a patient is at a low ebb, he will generally do the exercise with a vengeance for the first few days. One patient had strained his back severely, pushing a gas range onto a truck. He was a lugubrious man in his early forties, with a long history of back trouble and pessimism. I showed him the corrective exercise, and he couldn't believe it would work, though in his feeling of helplessness he was ready to try anything. "It's such a nothing exercise," he said.

I couldn't resist a pun: "Nothing ventured, nothing gained."

He got the idea, and really worked on correcting his back. I told him he could do the exercise as often as he liked. He did it every half hour, and by the third day his hip joint was beginning to stabilize. Two days later, maintaining the same pace, he was completely relieved. And two weeks later, he called to tell me he was doing fine. At this time, he expressed the fears he had been too frightened to voice.

"I was afraid the damn' thing would start all over again, and keep me crippled for months like it had once before. That's why I didn't get off my back for three days doing that exercise."

I was gratified by his fast recovery, particularly since fears and frustrations, suppressed or expressed, often create so much tension that resulting pressures keep the stressed joint slipping out. Muscular stress is directly related to emotional stress. One day, a weary-looking man in his late thirties limped in. I was struck more by the grimness of his expression than the list of his shoulder. He was so unhappy and depressed that he was loathe even to talk about his condition, other than to say his back was aching, and had been aching for years. He had the typical low-back syndrome, pain over the sacral area, pain shooting down one leg, a crooked back, and a shoulder you could roll marbles off of. But he was so sullen and uncommunicative that I thought something deep-seated must be bothering him. Perhaps he had lost his job, or his wife had left him, or he had suffered a heavy financial reverse. All these things happen all the time to people and I thought it might account for the funk he was in.

I decided to sit him down and have a heart to heart talk as I thought that speaking about his problems might make him feel better and at the same time relax him for the therapy. When I asked him a few leading questions, his face broke into a smile for the first time.

"Doctor," said he, "you have it all wrong. You are looking at a man with only one problem, and that's a bad back."

His story was a familiar one. He had taken his back to many medical offices and clinics. He had been told finally that he had a severe disc problem that would require surgery. He feared having the operation and feared not having it. His condition seemed to be getting progressively worse, and he was afraid that either way, surgery or gradual deterioration, he might wind up a cripple for the rest of his life.

I had to laugh at myself for not recognizing the depression syndrome so typical of a long-time sacroiliac. But I was able to reassure him, after a thorough examination, that his problems were mechanical and that he could put away his fears as his machine would soon be in good order. I lightly accentuated the positive. "I have had many cases like yours," I said, "and I have yet to lose a sacroiliac."

He breathed easier at the prospect of a correction without surgery. I put his sacroiliac in place, and showed him the corrective exercise. I told him to do it as often as he wanted at first, but no less than a dozen times a day, as I wanted him keeping his mind occupied with something productive. This was as good a way as any I knew of getting his mind and body to relax and to get him to stop feeling sorry for himself.

A week later his posture was already noticeably improved. But, more significantly, he was cheerful and completely at ease. Not once had the sacroiliac slipped out of joint, and the corrective exercise was not the only factor. Once he stopped worrying and relaxed, the tension in his lumbar muscles eased and his sacroiliac joint slid into place. He had learned to correct his emotional imbalance as well as his back.

I had him come in two weeks later, and the hip was still in place. Two weeks after that I discharged him as fully cured—emotionally and sacroiliacally, after recommending our rejuvenating exercises, which I outlined for him. Constant use of these exercises would do much to rebuild this man's physical and emotional stamina, eliminating the heavy stress patterns which had debilitated his personality.

There are very good physiological reasons for beneficial reactions to the proper stretch exercises. Exercise well-taken reduces the extreme adrenal stimulus produced under emotional excitation. This gives the individual in this flight-or-fight glandular situation an opportunity to keep his muscles relaxed and in repose. The adrenals under emotional stress—fear, resentment, anger—respond naturally to a jungle-type situation. But "civilized" man tries to keep cool and calm, not moving impulsively in any direction. And in standing quiet, while the stress is boiling up inside, the individual's adrenals become overtaxed as they are aborted in their normal function to activate bone, muscles, ligaments into an integrated striking force.

Exercise takes up the slack in an emotional crisis. If a person is angry and gets down on the floor and begins bending, twisting and flexing there will be an immediate —if temporary—relaxation of mind and body. The adrenalins become involved in this sublimated response of physical and mental stimuli, and the individual begins to simmer down. When the muscle is tensed for action and no action results, then the muscles stay tense and contracted. Unless he works off this tension, the person may make a sudden move, and displace a sacroiliac which is reacting to the tension in him.

Even when not fully conscious of his own emotional tension, suppressed for reasons of his own, the individual is still subject to the tensions they impose subconsciously. Many people looking for easy relaxation are often hoisted on their own petard as their search for pleasure jars a deep inner chord. I have nothing against sex, and, like the ancient Romans, feel it can be a constructive exercise between two consenting adults with no other attachments. But when a married man or woman deliberately ventures into a sexual excursion with somebody else, he or she is asking for trouble, and I don't mean legally or morally, as that is outside my province. In cheating on an unsuspecting partner, the faithless spouse is more likely to have a heart attack than at any other time. He is anything but relaxed inside, subconsciously he is ridden by feelings of guilt. Consequently, there is a great deal of nerve and muscular tension that ordinarily wouldn't manifest itself. His heart is pounding faster than it would normally in these circumstances—and that could be quite some pounding—and his whole system is being set up for anything he is particularly vulnerable to. If his heart is a weak spot, he may have a heart attack; if it's his back, his sacroiliac may slip out. In most instances of sex resulting in coronaries, statistics show the victim of such an attack has been participating in extra-marital sex, while the absent partner thinks his dearly beloved is engaged elsewhere in some innocent pursuit.

This is a very interesting commentary on American morals and mores, one, I hope, which will influence couples to enjoy a wonderful natural function without deception, in the relaxed embrace of their lawful partner, knowing they are where they properly belong. In this way, the old Roman exercise will be preserved in all its fidelity, and all that begins well will end well.

CHAPTER VII

Back Headaches

He had been having the severest headaches it had ever been my dubious privilege to observe.

He was an accountant, in his early thirties, and he had a history of bad headaches. The last was so severe that he couldn't think, eat, sleep, or work. He was taken to the hospital, and put on pain pills while various tests were made—X rays, neurological reflex tests, etc. There were no signs of any pathology as far as these tests were concerned. They were preparing to do an encephalogram that might confirm the possibility of a tumor in the brain, when some relatives, who were patients of mine, suggested that he try my approach. He agreed, and at his insistence was referred to me from the hospital.

He was a little hazy with pain killers when he came to me. But the pain still broke through the sedation, and his eyes were glazed with suffering. He was constantly nauseated, and did not feel able to go anywhere alone. He was in a bad way.

I checked his reflexes and general condition, and found these normal. In fact, everything checked normally, except for the spine. Checking his spine, I found a typical scoliotic pattern, a typical tilted pelvis pattern, and a typical tenderness at the base of the skull. This suboccipital area was very painful to the touch, as was the second cervical in the neck. From my point of view he had enough symptoms in this critical region to warrant the trouble he had been having.

My first procedure was to correct the sacroiliac joint. I showed him the corrective exercise but he was in such a drugged condition that he couldn't follow my directions. Not till the third visit was his head clear enough to understand this simple exercise.

His lower back had been out so long that it took several treatments on my part before the sacroiliac showed signs of stabilizing. By this time the pain in the neck was no longer constant but intermittent and we were able to cut down on the drugs. In the hospital, the pain had been so unremitting that they had given him codeine and morphine, drugs certainly not to be played around with. I took him off these and, meanwhile, used ice packs to reduce the stress to the suboccipital bone. Gradually, after three weeks, as the sacroiliac joints became stable and the spine began to relax, the headaches disappeared.

The corrective exercise was tremendously helpful. He did this at home after the first week, and it straightened out his scoliosis once the sacroiliac stayed in place. As for his remaining drugs, I tapered these off, and at the end of two weeks he was off them completely—for the first time in years.

Now that he was relaxed and out of pain, I showed him the neck rolls to keep his neck muscles flexible and strong, and I advised other rejuvenating exercises to get motion in the spine, while making sure the sacroiliac stayed in place.

The headaches seem to have permanently disappeared. He is back on his job, pursuing his sedentary course, and as long as he pursues his exercises with equal vigor, I have no expectation of seeing him back in my office.

In chronic headaches, I do not exclude the possibility that even where there is a spinal misalignment there may be some other factor contributing to the problem. Shortly after I worked out the corrective exercise technique, a young lady came in complaining of constant headaches. They were so severe that she couldn't drive her car more than ten or fifteen miles at a time as the jouncing over the highways aggravated the dull ache already there. I could tell looking from the way she listed to one side as she walked in that she probably had a sacroiliac displacement, but I proceeded to give her a complete physical examination. I checked her eyes, and made sure that she had been checked over recently by a reputable oculist. Actually she had recently had a thorough eye examination, and her vision was twenty-twenty, well-nigh perfect, without any astigmatic strain. Her blood pressure was good, her general reflexes normal. Various urine and blood samples revealed only that she was constitutionally a very sound young lady. Her skin was clear, and her nutritional habits excellent. As far as I could see, she had nothing wrong but an acute scoliosis. Yet, at the age of twenty-five, she had been suffering for years from agonizing neck pains and headaches. I felt that these were only symptoms.

Her family had persuaded her to visit me. She lived

125 miles north of Los Angeles, working as a secretary, and she had recently broken off regular weekend visits to her parents' home because of the jarring discomfort involved in driving that distance. She had come in to see me only to satisfy them. And she had a headache when she arrived.

She seemed amused by my preoccupation with an area so apparently remote from her problem. Although there were scoliotic curves in both the neck and dorsal vertebrae, I did not manipulate any part of the spine except the sacroiliac. I had no way of knowing how long the sacroiliac had been out. But her discomfort had begun when she was nineteen, and since she was now twenty-five, it was safe to say that the condition had commenced six years before, constantly aggravated with time and mounting stress.

At any rate, I adjusted her sacroiliac, and told her about the corrective exercise. Since it would take two or three weeks to stabilize a joint that had been out so long, the corrective exercise which could be done anywhere, was a double blessing for this out-of-town case. She checked in with me every ten days or so, and began to show marked improvement on her third visit. She is now back to normal, free of her headaches, and I haven't seen her for some time, though I do get occasional favorable reports from her parents, who are grateful that their daughter is able to visit them regularly again.

Time and again, I have received confirmation that if the cause is corrected, the apparent secondary effects—headaches, sciatica, scoliotic curvature—will disappear as a matter of course.

Many nagging headaches are the result of stress patterns involving the muscles attached to the suboccipital bone. If the patient moves his fingers along the back of his head at the base of the skull where these muscles attach, he will find this area highly sensitive to the touch, indicating inflammation at this point. Because of nerve patterns, the pain stimuli from suboccipital stress travels along one side of the head or may encompass both sides.

Mental tension is a factor in these spinal-oriented headaches, since additional tension precipitates a tightening effect on neck and upper dorsal muscles already under stress from the sacroiliac displacement. And it has an irritating action at the place where the spine meets the skull because of the muscle attachments at that point pulling on the bone. Because of the sensitivity of this area, with all the nerve pathways radiating in every direction, it would be surprising if the afflicted individual didn't have a headache problem. The pain in these cases usually comes from a stress point at the suboccipital bone which tends to overstimulate the nerves. Remove the stress and you remove the pain. And this holds true in eighty percent of the headaches cases brought to my attention.

Some headache sufferers have had these stress patterns for so long that the inflammation at the suboccipital bone has become chronic and extra help is needed to reverse the headache syndrome. In exceptionally stubborn cases, I recommend inverted exercises such as the headstand or the shoulder stand, if the headstand presents any problems. These inverted postures increase the circulation to the inflamed neck area, accelerating the healing process already instigated by the replacement of the sacroiliac. Of course the corrective exercises help too.

At the outset, the patient should stay in the shoulder stand or headstand position for no more than a minute, gradually increasing to four or five minutes. By stimulating the circulatory response in the neck area, you carry away harmful toxins and reduce pain and irritation as you reduce toxicity.

The shoulder stand, easier for the novice to maintain, is especially helpful, as muscle strain of the neck is relaxed and these muscles beneficially stretched, relieving tension at the suboccipital bone. You should feel comfortable not only in doing the shoulder stand, but in all other exercises described in this book. Otherwise, you are defeating the main purpose, for you may overextend yourself, and only succeed in aggravating the original strain. Especially where there has been an injury, one should begin cautiously and gradually step up the pace. If an exercise is painful, this is nature's warning that you are overdoing, so ease up. It doesn't always follow that if a little of something is good that a lot is better. But if the exercises are done judiciously, and the spine is kept in alignment, headache relief should be lasting. Unfortunately, the chronic patient often forgets as the headaches leave him how painful they were, and how he was helped. He lazily drifts out of the exercise habit and the neck muscles begin to tighten up again, even though the spine is aligned. There may even be a resurgence of the old familiar headaches. The wise patient will continue whatever helped him, including the head and neck rolls, which maintain good postural control of the neck. Just make a full rotation to the left and then right, three times for each, slowly, comfortably, without strain or pain. When you hear those clicks in your neck, be assured that you are wearing down trouble-making calcium deposits. In doing this exercise, a proper breathing pattern will help to time the exercise properly and control the motion. In this way, you take in helpful oxygen while establishing a perfect rhythmical pattern so essential to relaxation.

Perhaps because of emotional problems, the young seem at least as susceptible to headache problems as their elders. An eighteen-year-old patient, a slim, lovely model, complained to me of severe headaches. They had been troubling her for months. I gave her the usual checkout, which was negative. She was a very healthy specimen over-all, and then I checked her spine and pelvic area. Both sacroiliac joints were badly displaced. I corrected her myself, then showed her the corrective exercise and told her to follow through at home, every hour or so if possible, since the displacement was so bad that it had twisted her spine into a complete lateral curvature, with the tension clearly apparent to the touch in the suboccipital region. She felt immediate relief from my adjustment. But the muscle tension was so great that her sacroiliac practically slipped out by itself that night. She called me the next morning, and I told her to do the exercise I had shown her. She had realized her sacroiliac was out again when that new feeling of freedom left her lower back area. This set up a chain reaction which resulted in her headache returning.

She wanted to come in and see me again, but I told her that I could not do anything more than she could do for herself with the exercise I had shown her. She found it hard to believe that she could help herself with so simple a procedure, and admitted she hadn't done the exercise. I then told her to come in the following day, as I wanted her to build up her confidence in her power to help herself. I also wanted to make sure that she was doing the exercise properly.

She came in the next day, and I could tell from her relaxed and carefree air that the exercise was working. The low-back pressure had disappeared, she was walking on air, and the headache was gone.

"I just can't believe it," she said.

She had done the exercise perfectly, her hips and pubic bones were absolutely even, the distortion in her spine was easing, and the tenderness in the suboccipital area had diminished greatly, all in forty-eight hours.

I showed her some of our Yoga-type exercises, told her they would have aesthetic advantages, as well as being physically beneficial, and she is now doing them faithfully. I only hear of her now from her mother, who is also a patient.

I have had people come in with lifts in their shoes, who are still troubled with backache—and headache. As I have mentioned elsewhere I am against lifts, as they only fix the degree of error or displacement. To be sure, if the lift is correctly measured to the amount of displacement, it may help a scoliotic problem for a time. But unfortunately for the lift-wearer, when the degree of displacement changes, as it is prone to do, the spine forms a new compensating curve. Even worse, if the sacroiliac joint should resume its normal position through a fortuitous movement, the lift would force the spine into a lateral curvature to compensate for this newly artificially induced tilt of the pelvis. So actually, a lift should never be used unless there is a true short leg and the lift brings both ilial bones in their proper apposition to the sacrum.

One headache patient with a lift also had a vomiting problem. Many times a patient with a sacroiliac displacement will have a vomiting reflex along with headaches. Vomiting is also related to other ailments, such as cranial tumor, which could also cause headaches. Before sending her off to a neurologist, I thought I would do what I could to relieve her, always keeping it in mind that she might have a brain tumor.

The first thing I did was measure her legs, separately and together. She did not have a true short leg. I removed the lift from her shoe, and slipped both sacroiliac joints back in place. Then I showed her the corrective exercise. She seemed tremendously relieved, and the vomiting urge almost immediately subsided. I looked for and found muscle tension in the suboccipital area. I was convinced we were on the right track, but I wanted her back for another checkup. On her return two days later, she seemed a new woman. The headaches had disappeared, and so had the nausea. I told her to continue the corrective exercise, making it part of a lifelong routine, and to throw away the lift. She would never need it again—and she never has.

Our most dramatic success has come from migraine headaches. Migraines are usually on one side of the head, in the temporal (temple) area. It is a miserable affliction. The patient, in agonizing pain, feels an almost uncontrollable impulse to bang his head against a wall.

Quite often, the pain is so severe that nausea is common. Usually, the victim has a warning feeling that an attack is coming, and may turn to a drug, a course I don't advocate. There is a definite neurological syndrome to migraine. If you look closely at the blood vessels on the affected side of the head, you'll find they are often swollen and distended because of a congested reaction to tension. The tension centers in the back of the neck, and head, at the point of the suboccipital bone. If you remove the pressure from the suboccipital, you automatically relieve the muscle pull on this bone, easing the inflammation at the base of the skull. In this way, you will nearly always correct a migraine headache.

The displaced sacroiliac is basically one of the major causes for stress to the back of the neck and head. You nearly always will have a displaced sacroiliac with a migraine. And you always have a scoliosis, indicating that the stress is transferred directly from the lateral curvature in the dorsal spine to the upper cervicals in the neck. When a vasomotor situation is consequently created through somatic change, the motor nerves in that particular vascular or circulatory area are stimulated in such a way that they change the size of the blood vessels, accentuating the pressures in the cranial area. There is invariably an emotional trigger touching off every migraine, a job upset, a family quarrel, anger, or fear. The syndrome, the scoliosis and suboccipital tightness, is already present and ready to be triggered. At a moment's notice, the nerve stimulus sets off the chain reaction that almost drives the sufferer out of his mind with pain. It just didn't happen in one day. Behind every migraine are

years of stress which made the victim especially susceptible to vasomotor stimulus at this impressionable base of
the skull area.

People with migraines tend to be emotional people.
Seldom are they the placid type. The disorder makes no
distinction of age or sex. They are all ages, and as many
men seem affected as women, which is rather odd, since
women are considered the more emotional. Usually, as
with a thirty-year-old housewife, they have a long history
of spinal problems. This woman had an unstable sacroiliac, a pronounced scoliosis, and fortunately, a good
sense of humor. While I was checking her hipbones, she
quipped through gritted teeth:

"That's not what's aching."

She was one of those chronic sacroiliacs whose body
had inured itself to the original injury, and was picking
up the pain stimuli from a subsidiary stress area in the
upper spine.

Tension in the suboccipital area, the telltale symptom,
was plainly apparent to the touch, and it was from this
area the blinding pain was emanating. The stress on the
suboccipital bone had as long a history as her headaches.
And since she had suffered these headaches for years, it
would take weeks and months of constant correction perhaps for the spine to regain a normal curvature with absolute comfort at the suboccipital bone.

I told her all this as I corrected her sacroiliac, and
showed her the corrective exercise. As I said, she was a
typical migrainer. She looked at me sharply, as if upset
by my forecast of the course of her malady.

"You're not very optimistic," she said.

"You will get better gradually," I told her, "and the severity and number of the headaches will diminish until one day, with muscles—and mind—perfectly relaxed, your migraines will disappear."

She gave a grunt of satisfaction.

"Don't let anything upset you," I said.

Even this mild enjoinder seemed to set her off.

"How can you help it if people are unkind to you?" she said tartly.

I sighed inwardly. "Just remember that when you let anything upset you, you only hurt yourself."

After she left, I found myself thinking that her spine might very well straighten up one day—but there was very little I could do about her mind. She would have to straighten that out herself.

CHAPTER VIII

Of Discs and Whiplash

The discs are the body's shock absorbers.

As we get older, these hardy cushions of cartilage be-tween the spinal vertebrae tend to degenerate and break down with time, use, scoliotic change, and trauma. As these pads deteriorate and wear thin, individuals may lose a half-inch, inch, even an inch and a half in height. In some instances, a patient will come in and complain he's lost as much as two inches in height—usually as the small pads of cartilage between the vertebrae lose density through shrinkage or attribution. You could lose less than an eighth of an inch in each of the twenty-four spinal discs, and still lose more than two inches.

Because of gravitation, there is a constant downward pressure on the discs from the fact that our trunks are usually in an upright position, sitting or standing. This pressure is relieved in the horizontal position, lying down. And there are exercises, outlined in the appendix, which stretch the spine, keeping it flexible, and help the sensitive pads between the vertebrae retain their original resilience and function.

The Cobra, a Yoga exercise, and the various supine exercises we recommend have a tendency to stretch the inner spaces and the ligament attachments of the vertebrae, giving the discs more latitude of movement while easing gravitational pressures. At the same time, they are keeping these discs flexible, retarding the shrinking process so that the middle-aged not only keep their youthful tallness but even gain some height in the process.

A growing number of backaches concern so-called disc problems. I say so-called because the only true disc problem in my experience involves an herniation of the disc, where the disc itself ruptures and presses agonizingly on a nerve trunk issuing out of the spinal cord. This poses a severe problem marked by acute pain, some loss of muscle function. Unless all these things apply, I do not consider it a herniated disc problem. With herniation, the patient may be unable to move a leg because he lacks motor-nerve control. In this event, a neurologist should be consulted to probe the nature of the pressure from the herniated disc. He may have to perform necessary surgery. However, much of the surgery on the back is not only unnecessary but dangerous. Often, when there is an unexplained back problem of a recurring nature, surgery is performed to fuse two or more vertebrae together without taking into account a long-standing sacroiliac displacement which very likely is the cause of the recurring problem.

In these fusions, to compensate for aging or traumatized discs, two or more vertebrae are fused together, connected by a transplanted piece of bone, to make one solid vertebra. The offending disc is usually removed, as by removing motion stress in that area the pain is removed or reduced. You lose flexibility at this point, but enough vertebrae are functioning to maintain a certain limited flexibility.

Fusion surgery is frequently a spectacular failure. Actor Jeff Chandler succumbed in the hospital after lower-back surgery, and President John F. Kennedy kept his bad back until the day he was assassinated. After the President's fusion operation, he continued to suffer pain along with a loss of flexibility. If the pain was due to some other pathology, such as a sacroiliac misalignment, then fusion wouldn't solve the problem. And it didn't.

Where a disc problem is suspected, and the surgeon removes the disc, the body usually fills in the gap with fibrous tissue, and the patient, if lucky, may be little the worse for the experience. But dangerous complications can be avoided if the sacroiliac is checked out and properly given the blame. Disc surgery side effects can be horrendous—paralysis, hemorrhage, infection, overgrowth of fibrous tissue. Often surgeons have to go back and clean out an infection or remove fibrous excess.

Some orthopedic men are gradually cutting down on surgery, and leaning to more conservative techniques. In England, under anesthesia and with the help of a myelogram, an X ray indicating the disc herniation in the spine, there have been successful efforts to manipulate the disc back through the herniated opening and relieve pressure on the nerve trunk. In one case, I was able to use this technique myself, without relying on a myelogram, just by judging the sensitivity of the involved area under my fingers. Through manipulation I returned the disc to its proper place, relieving the pressure and the pain which had resulted when the disc pressed against the delicate membrane of the nerve trunk.

It was a ticklish procedure. There was a partial paralysis of the left leg. This was particularly disturbing as the patient was a mailman, and unable to perform his duties. He was helped into my office by a friend. There was considerable pain in the leg, and he was unable to lift it or change its position. It had all the appearance of a truly herniated disc. I deemed it advisable to send him to a neurologist for a consultation and a myelogram. But I decided, having studied the remanipulating technique, that I would give it a try. There was certainly nothing to lose. I put him on the treatment table, examined him carefully, checked out the spine level at which the disc appeared herniated, and proceeded to manipulate the affected disc into its original position. It is a very difficult procedure, as one has to sense correctly just how much motion can be applied to the vertebrae and in which direction. In rotating the spinal bones in this way, there is an almost immediate cessation of pain, as the disc is eased away from the nerve trunk. Meanwhile, correcting the ilial bones below, I altered the position of the spinal column, giving the crooked spine a chance to normalize.

Seldom have I seen a "slipped disc" where there hasn't been a sacroiliac displacement. This basic malposition and the scoliotic changes in the spine above induce the pressure which causes the disc to lose shape and herniate when outside stresses occur. So we treat the cause as well as the symptoms. In the case of the mailman, I was able to get results, taking pressure off the nerves involved and returning the control of his leg to him.

As time goes on, the scoliotic curve produces stresses on discs as well as vertebrae. If the spine is straight, each vertebra and disc pressing down normally, the pressure is evened out, and the possibility of herniation minimized. But if the spine has a compound tilt, tilting sideways as well as forward and backward, the disc at this curvature point is pressed with such thrust that it may form a bubble or nipple, and it is this protruding tissue which now presses on the nerve trunk.

There is no doubt in my mind, after observing literally thousands of cases, that endless irritation of the vertebrae through constant compression, causing cartilage and bone to rub against each other, tends to stimulate calcium spurs along the edges of the bone, producing arthritis of the spine.

Discs don't rupture without reason. Usually they are spread thin by time and attrition, ready for a triggering event. Most true disc injuries occur when the patient is bending forward, as in making a bed. In the lumbar, lower spine, the anterior or frontal density of the disc is usually higher than the posterior density. In bending forward the edge with the higher density is compressed with resulting pressure on the thinner posterior edge of the disc and the rupture occurs. There is no actual slippage. The disc is merely pressed down against the nerve trunk. Actually, unless it breaks through the protective membrane of the spinal cord, the herniated disc may never bother the individual. In a recent hospital survey, two hundred spinal autopsies on patients without any back history revealed numerous herniated discs, which the patients didn't even know they had, because there was no pressure on the nerve trunk and no pain.

As with any ailment, it is far better to avoid it than treat it. Applying the corrective exercise and certain rejuvenating exercises, we keep the spine straight and strong, the discs flexible and even, and the "slipped disc" problem magically disappears, even where the vertebrae have formed calcium deposits (unless it is a true herniation).

The mechanics of spinal health are quite simple. With the alignment of the pelvic bone or hipbone, the vertebrae above the sacrum now rebalance and re-form in a normal narrow single S curve, instead of a compound scoliotic curve where the figure S curves laterally up the spine. With the scoliosis removed, the spine relaxed, the disc's normal position and density is automatically re-established sooner or later. The likelihood of a herniated disc is virtually nonexistent in these circumstances. Once the disc is in proper alignment, the downward gravity pull that distorts the disc in a crooked spine has no adverse effect as the pressure is modified or counteracted by this even distribution. In my experience, it is only when the disc is squeezed out of its normal shape and position by spinal misalignment that there is a related disc injury. Otherwise, aside from accidents, there is little chance of injuring the disc. Invariably, in so-called disc complaints I look for and find a displaced sacroiliac and scoliotic curvature of the spine.

Even when the disc condition has prevailed for months and the disc has narrowed, as long as there is natural resilience in the body, the disc will tend to normalize with an alignment of the sacroiliac. Even flattened down at an angle, the disc by virtue of its semi-soft, pliant consistency will resume its original alignment and density, freed of pressure.

With the average "slipped disc," apart again from a herniated or ruptured disc, the pain is not related to the disc but to muscle spasms and strained ligaments in the lumbar and dorsal spine—these directly related to the displaced sacroiliac joint.

For this reason I am opposed to fusion operations, as my experience shows that practically all lower-back problems can be resolved, with that one exception mentioned above, by correction of the sacroiliac joints and mobilization of the lumbar spine through removing spasms and tensions with our rejuvenating exercises.

Actually, even the truly herniated disc is related to the sacroiliac. For there is no herniated disc in my experience without a displaced sacroiliac. The herniation occurs either at the time that the sacroiliac is displaced—generally a very traumatic displacement—or it could result from an accumulation of spinal stress induced by a severe pelvic tilt.

I nearly always shudder when I hear that somebody has had a fusion. As a rule, it is not only unnecessary but only serves to reduce the flexibility of the spine, without, I repeat, getting at the cause. Fortunately, fusions are falling out of fashion, as word of mouth is making patients more aware of its dangers and ineffectiveness.

Still, patients are forever hobbling in with what they call disc problems. So long as they have not had spinal fusions there is a good chance they can be relieved of

their problem. The wife of a Los Angeles attorney was referred to me with a "disc" problem after she had been
treated at a reputable clinic for nine months. She had
been hospitalized with traction, given heat packs (the
worst thing for her), and then fitted with a brace or supporting corset about her lower waist and hips. With it all
she was still in pain, and partially immobilized, hard-
pressed to attend to the small child that she had to daily
lift in and out of its crib and play pen. She was then told
that surgery was the only thing that could possibly help
her. Rather than submit to that, she consulted me. I had
her remove the brace so I could examine her properly.
Sure enough, she had a decided pelvic tilt, and her sacroiliac was obviously displaced. I could see the displacement from across the room. I corrected the displacement, showed her the corrective exercise, and suggested
she come in two or three times in the next two weeks,
meanwhile doing the exercise at home. She could hardly
believe that the problem which had begun to dominate
her life could be so simply resolved. But she was encour-
aged by the immediate results gained from putting back
the sacroiliac joint. She was able to walk out of the office,
without the corset and with comparatively little pain.
After she did the exercise for a few weeks, stabilizing
the sacroiliac joint's balance and alignment, she gradually
improved until she was virtually one hundred percent
better. She was in such good shape, alas, that she became
careless one day, and while shopping lifted a heavy bag
better left to her husband. She was in a panic, thinking
she might have started the whole problem all over again.
But there was no need for concern. She had re-established

the strain, pulling her sacroiliac out, but it was not quite as severe, as the corrective exercise had strengthened her lower-back area. The sacroiliac was put back in place, she returned to the corrective exercise several times a day, and two weeks later she was totally relieved, able to twist, bend, or lift, as every healthy person should be able to do. Today, if she feels the slightest twinge or ache in the lower-back area, she immediately does the corrective exercise, and is promptly relieved. She was very depressed emotionally when she first came to me, wondering at the age of thirty whether she would ever be able to adequately discharge her family obligations to her husband and her child. Today, she is a supremely confident young lady, very capably handling every domestic duty that comes her way. As for the brace, that went the way of her slipped disc—into oblivion.

Backache and automobile accidents seem to go together. And there must be several hundred thousand accidents a year.

Anybody who has been backended by another car knows how traumatic a whiplash injury can be. The neck and shoulder muscles may remain stiff and sore for months, even years, unless proper corrective action is promptly taken. In order to treat the whiplash effectively, it is important to know exactly what happens to the neck when, in the jar of the collision, it snaps back without warning.

When whiplash occurs, the ligaments holding the cervical vertebrae in their normal apposition are stretched suddenly, and certain dorsal and lumbar vertebrae and the sacroiliac joint itself may also be pulled out of alignment.

Often this is not spotted by the therapist and consequently the low-back area receives no treatment.

The accident—and injury—happens so rapidly that nature has no opportunity to form a protective mechanism to modify the damage. The trauma is much like a bad ankle sprain. There is a rupturing of the tissue, a tearing of minute blood vessels, an abrupt extension of ligaments and tendons beyond their normal elasticity—and muscle spasms with a certain amount of swelling.

Often, no treatment is given for the swelling, though ice packs would beneficially reduce it in two or three days. The swelling, interfering with the healing process, keeps the tissues stretched beyond normal for an extended period, and the neck may remain troublesome for years—or forever. It is the same with an ankle sprain. By immediately packing that ankle in ice, the swelling is reduced to an absolute minimum in two or three days, and the overstretching is accordingly reduced. With this reduction there is less work for the body to do in bringing these traumatized tissues back to normal strength, and the ankle may be perfectly normal in two or three weeks. And the same would be true of the neck, if the injury were immediately detraumatized, giving the tissues a chance to heal, and the sacroiliac were adjusted, giving the overextended ligaments in the spine a chance to normalize.

Whiplash injury, however, is more complex than an ankle sprain. In the attempt to free the neck, and restore normal movement, one group of muscles have a tendency to pull or tighten up as you try to relax another group. If it is possible to get yourself in a completely relaxed position, and rotate the neck easily without antagonizing certain muscles, you may succeed in slipping everything into place.

We have a simple exercise for this procedure, the head and neck roll. If done while the rest of the body is perfectly relaxed, it will bring about a reduction of neck and shoulder tension.

But even with this exercise, it should be remembered that basically the sacroiliac is responsible for most of the tension in the neck. I have treated hundreds of whiplash cases. And almost without exception, I have found that the sacroiliac is displaced at the same time the cervical whiplash occurs. This is a major reason for the whiplash's notable resistance to purely localized treatment. In a pelvic tilt, with a scoliotic change in the spine, the curvature extends from the sacral bone to the base of the skull. And so it becomes obvious that if you treat the neck, without correcting the spinal curvature, you are not getting at the root of the problem. As a rule, even when I'm treating a person who has had a whiplash problem for two or three years, I can correct the sacroiliac joint quickly and see the patient get up and walk around freely in my office.

Many tell me that there is fifty percent more motion in their necks, although I haven't even touched their neck. If they were to do the corrective exercise, putting back their own sacroiliac joints, the result would be the same. If the whiplash injury has been prolonged, they may have to do the corrective exercise more frequently in the beginning, as the hipbone, at the bottom of all this, will slip back for a while before it finally stabilizes. It may take six weeks to establish a new spinal alignment in such chronic cases. With a much slacker joint, and a less recent injury, it may take three months. It may even take a year in cases where the back has been out of place twenty or thirty years. While the patient may get some instant relief, he will have to work at the exercise to keep feeling better.

Sometimes whiplash injuries are so severe that the victim takes to his or her bed. In one case, a lady was carted home from an auto accident and was incapable of leaving the house. She was a housewife in her midforties and she was totally incapacitated and in shock. I visited the home and checked her over. We had X rays made. They were negative for fracture, but the neck was swollen and extremely painful to the touch or the slightest movement. It even hurt her to get out of bed or walk. Other muscles, typical of a bad whiplash, were also affected, from the mastoid bone in the back of the ear to the sternum or breastbone. When the head snapped back, these muscles were severely strained and the patient was in constant pain, with severe headaches. Both sacroiliac joints were out and I corrected them, without recommending the corrective exercise at this time, as she just wouldn't have been able to get comfortable enough to do it. My first task, after the adjustment, was to get the swelling down. I ordered constant ice packs for seventy-two hours to reduce the edema, and thus improve blood flow to the wounded area. In a very severe whiplash, I sometimes prescribe a supporting collar as any unexpected roll or motion will additionally overextend already extended muscles. But in this case, since she was staying at home, not riding in a moving vehicle, or stepping off a curb, I didn't

see the necessity. And I generally prefer a certain freedom of motion, if it can be controlled. The ice did its job,
the swelling was quickly reduced, and the normalized
spine aided in the patient's progress. In three weeks she
was able to make it into my office unaided. The pain and
swelling were almost nonexistent. I showed her the corrective exercise, she executed it perfectly, and in a few more
weeks, she didn't even realize she had had a whiplash
injury. Had it not been for the ice pack's dramatic work,
and the sacroiliac correction, she would have been in for
at least a year's treatment. A severe whiplash is nothing
to be trifled with, and the result, a weak, tender neck,
sometimes remains for a lifetime. So always try to get at
the seat of a continuing whiplash problem. The sacroiliac
may get rid of that pain in your neck.

CHAPTER IX   *Staying Young—Rejuvenation*

There has probably been more nonsense written and spoken about staying young than any other subject. Since staying young implies staying able, virile, healthier, and attractive longer, there is hardly anybody over twenty-one that isn't interested in a program that will accomplish this feat. Some proponents of perpetual youth push improved nutrition, with emphasis on organically grown natural foods. Others put stress on meditation and inner peace. Still others advocate exercises, jogging, walking, swimming, Yoga, competitive sports.

My own feeling is that continued health and vitality depends on a physically oriented program stressing optimum circulation, assimilation, and elimination. Sensible eating habits are a part of this program, as one can hardly assimilate or eliminate well, if he is eating devitalized foods. On the other hand, the proper exercise routine will lead the individual to an improved diet, as his stimulated circulation and increased glandular activity will almost intuitively direct him to the healthful diet that his renewed tissues are now demanding. In other words, digestive juices, muscles, ligaments, bones and other body tissue are involuntarily sending out a message for the nutrients they need to turn time around and assume the tone and resilience of youth. With a relaxed body, it is infinitely easier to command a relaxed mind capable of both analytic thought and subconscious flights of imagination that open an exciting prospect of a universe whose mysteries we have hardly begun to scratch. With a sense of union with the universe, resulting from the quiet of meditation, we in turn gain the insight that permits us to initiate or maintain a regimen that allows us to enjoy the longer life our muscles have earned for us.

It all begins with circulation. If we improve the circulation to the brain and the head, for instance, we retard the onset of senility. We improve the vision, hearing, everything that has to do with the senses. By keeping the capillaries in the head well-nourished with blood, we keep them open and elastic, and inhibit the tendency to strokes as we get older. Even the hair beginning to thin out or recede after forty or fifty, begins to grow back (particularly with the Yoga-type inverted exercises) and even darker in some instances. Middle-aged vision, presbyopia, where a book has to be held at an increasing distance, is slowed up and reading becomes less of a strain. The flow of blood, slowed to the extremities with time, has been stepped up once again, and the nerves responsible for the impulses to the eyes, ears, hair roots, etc., are beginning to receive the stimulation they require to maintain their function.

In our exercises, we stimulate with increased circulation every part of the body. The glands are notably affected by this blood bath. In the pelvic area, the muscles are reconditioned and the gonads, the sex glands, automatically stimulated. By improving the tone of the thyroid, pituitary and adrenal glands, the semicircular canals of the ear, we increase the body's all-around balance, and discourage marginal ailments such as diabetes and hypoglycemia. We improve resistance to exhaustion, displace a tendency in older people to get dizzy, and step up sexual activity. Our walk is springier, we require less sleep, memory improves. We start thinking again optimistically of what we want to accomplish. We stop brooding about getting old and decrepit and stop thinking about age as a limitation.

None of this is theory, all is pragmatic. I have seen my patients work wonders with these exercises, and have done them myself for years. Where a man of fifty is beginning to show the aging process, not quite hearing the voices he once heard, not quite up to an evening out after dinner, he gradually begins to act and react like his old self. From the age of fifty, for the next fifteen, twenty, or twenty-five years, he may amaze his friends by going through life with all its stresses, with little apparent change. The clock is truly turned back. Many men, as they get older, become concerned about their sexual activity, using this as a yardstick of their declining powers. This decline is largely a loss in vitality and a programed mental attitude. There is no limit to how old a man—or woman—can be for continued sexual activity. And he soon finds out with our exercises that sex has as much functional relationship to the body as breathing or sleeping. It is limited only by the diminished vitality of his endocrine system and his all-around physical prowess. With the exercises I advocate, the spine stays supple. We twist, turn, flex, change positions. Our joints stay limber, we bend our knees, our elbows, move our shoulders, extend our arms, twist our neck, do all the things that are necessary to function and be a viable young individual with viable glands and muscles.

It is remarkable what we can do once we accept the fact that we don't have to get old at a certain age. Starting at age forty-five and fifty, I have seen men pitch into these exercises and in two or three years, working out moderately every day, exceed the activity of a young man of twenty-five or thirty years who has not exercised for five or ten years.

Aging is a matter of metabolism. The body functions better as it gets rid of the toxic byproducts of metabolism before they build up into a toxemia often expressing itself as a degenerative disease. Somebody once said that the best route to a ripe old age is to pick the right grandparents. There is no question the genetic factor has a lot to do with the business of being youthful. However, we can modify this factor by the food we eat, the exercises we do, the thoughts we think, the toxins we breathe in, and the way we eliminate. In the same families, a differing mode of life is constantly expressed in a different aging process, though the genetic factors are obviously similar.

Two of my patients are brothers, one year apart. At the ages of fifty-four and fifty-five, they look more like father and son. And, more importantly, physically and mentally, the difference is even greater. The younger brother not only looks fifteen or twenty years older but, physically and mentally, is that much older as well. Only in their exercise routines has there been any great difference in living habits.

Both have pretty much the same eating habits, are in similar sedentary occupations, and have had a comparable domestic life, married and divorced. But whereas one practiced the Yoga-type exercises from the time he was forty, the other did nothing to counter certain genetic weaknesses that both had. At forty-five, because of a family tendency to deafness through aural nerve deterioration, the younger man started to lose his hearing. The older, through standing on his head and doing the shoulder stand, was able to resist this genetic susceptibility, and indeed improved his hearing. The younger had an early loss of hair, not unusual on the male side of his family. The other, in his midfifties, had a shock of hair as thick and bristly as it was in his twenties. His complexion was clear and crisp, his face ruddy and healthy looking, his eyes bright. He was seldom if ever tired, and never ill, except for a rare cold. The other brother, who disdained exercise as if it were the plague, was troubled by a bad back before he came to me, complained of chronic fatigue, looked and acted tired at all times. But most striking was the difference in the bearing of the two men.

The one who exercised had the posture of a young man, and moved with a young man's decision, energy and rhythm. The other just poked along uncertainly, his shoulders in a slouch, his body unco-ordinated, his head drooping. Mentally, too, there was a vast difference. The younger-but-older brother lived in the past, talking of the good old times. The other was constantly full of his plans for the day and the morrow. He had neither the time nor the inclination to reminisce. He was in the company of young, vital people at all times, communicating with them on their own level.

The other brother preferred, or needed, regular rest periods to recover from the business functions that he once handled with ease. Even so, with all his disabilities and malfunctions, it was not too late for him to get started on an exercise routine that would reverse the clock. But staying young, like getting old, begins in the head, and I could not get it through his head that he was still young enough, with a good enough constitution, to settle down into an exercise pattern that would restore his sagging vitality. I could do nothing with him. Mentally, he had accepted growing old, and was subconsciously looking forward to this state as a surcease from the struggles and sorrows that one is in constant contention with in the arena of life.

Meanwhile, the older of the two, I confidently predict, will be as active, as aggressively youthful, fifteen or twenty years from now as he is today, so long as he continues to exercise faithfully every day.

Time after time, I have seen what these daily exercises, with the corrective exercise thrown in, can do for patients who have come in with the variety of complaints common to the ordinary aging process. Just keeping the joints loose and limber, extending and improving the motion of the ligaments, not only keeps the individual moving around energetically, but reduces the calcium deposits which form in and around the joints due to inflammation and age. I have seen severe bursitis cases completely cured after several months of gradually increasing exercises, the calcium disappearing through absorption as the circulation to the area increases. In the same way bony spurs that have formed on the vertebrae have vanished with the mobilization of maximum motion in the spine, through insistent stretching, flexing, twisting and turning.

In these exercises, every part of the body is thoroughly massaged, including the viscera, which ordinarily receive very little stimulation, just sagging a little bit more and more with time as a result of the downward pull of gravitation. But with our exercises, bending, stretching, and inverting as we do, we bring increased circulation to the liver, pancreas, stomach, spleen, intestinal tract, the kidneys, all the viscera, and every part of the body. With this increased circulation, we excite changes in the tone of the male prostate and testicles, and the ovaries of the female. At the same time, because of increased circulatory activity, we hasten the metabolic process by breaking down and eliminating the cellular refuse which causes our aches and pains when we do anything unaccustomed as we get older. The efficiency with which the tissues dispose of waste—and with which they heal—are excellent indicators of the shape a person is in. I have known men of fifty-five, who healed faster than those of thirty-five or forty. Invariably, the quick healers were daily exercisers, and the younger men were sedentary creatures whose major exercise entailed opening and shutting the refrigerator door.

Somebody once said that the best exercise for sex is sex. I don't quite hold with that. However, I have found that exercises bearing directly on the organs you are specifically trying to activate usually are more immediately effective than exercises helping the body generally. The Shoulder Stand and the Plough, in which the legs are brought back stiffened over the head, are considered beneficial to the sex potential because of their stimulatory action on the thyroid gland in the notch of the throat. But for direct improvement in the sexual area, I favor exercises which directly strengthen and tone the organs in the pelvic area. I advocate exercises which involve the hips moving up and down and leg lifts which put a stress on the lower abdomen. I have not known anybody, regardless of age, who has been doing these exercises daily who is not able to function well sexually. As long as a man or woman maintains circulation and tone, they will maintain their sexual ability until the day nature sees fit to take them to their Maker.

The legs, anatomically farthest from the pumping action of the heart, are generally the first barometer of declining vigor. We see this clearly with athletes who depend more on their leg power for a livelihood than other people. With fighters, traditionally, the legs are the first to go, which is why road work is of paramount importance with those who square off against each other in the ring. By twenty-eight or thirty, with a changing metabolism, the fighter's legs have started to go, even though his shoulders and arms are as strong as ever. He must keep running, jogging, walking, to enable his legs to carry him through the grueling pace fighters have to maintain. After a long layoff, the erstwhile heavyweight champion, Cassius Clay (Muhammad Ali), fought flat-footed after three or four rounds, his legs no longer strong enough to keep him on his toes for fifteen rounds.

With ordinary folks, the demands are less, but the concept is the same. The circulation obviously improves the muscle tone. And the improved muscle tone in turn improves the circulation. Leg strength is dependent on the circulation to the legs. But then the blood traveling back to the heart has to be pushed up from the veins in the legs primarily by the muscular action of the legs, pushing the blood from this area into the central circulatory system. People with slightly swollen ankles often reduce the swelling with a long brisk walk, the leg muscles expanding and contracting into an action by which the blood is pushed back and drained from the extremities and the ankles begin to lose their edema. Now this interchange is true of practically all of the muscle tissues in the body. The more you use your muscles, the more you are able to improve the circulation, bathing the tissues with life-renewing blood that retards the aging process as long as it is humanly possible.

Like the legs, the head is another extremity which suffers first from circulatory problems because the heart muscles have a greater distance to push the blood. And so as the heart loses some of its youthful vigor, circulation diminishes to the head as well as the legs. Senility, which everyone dreads, reflects a gradual loss of circulation to the cells of the brain, with a resulting loss of capillary tone and function. With increased circulation, function is always improved. In emphysema, for instance, as we deep-breathe, even with a certain amount of damage to the lungs, we are using parts of the lung we haven't been using before. The same holds true with arthritis. By bringing the affected joints into easy and gradual motion, we increase circulation and enhance the ability of the bones to move in correspondence with the controlling ligaments and tendons. Function is directly related to the motion you convey to tissue. The more motion, the more function, and the more function, the more motion.

With our exercises, elimination is noticeably improved, diminishing toxics and lessening the likelihood of a general toxemia predisposing the individual to illness and breakdowns. By improving cell efficiency, we draw the excess water from the tissues, and squeeze the fluid out of the system. Invariably, after a half hour of these exercises, the exerciser visits the bathroom. The pressure exerted by the various stretching and bending movements seems to increase the ability of the kidneys and its tubules to pick up fluid and eliminate it promptly through the kidneys and the bladder. With less fluid retention, the tone of the tissues improve and so does its function. The whole economy of the system is improved, with improved assimilation, circulation, and elimination.

Your body, using oxygen more efficiently, utilizes it as a source of greater energy. Additionally, the food you eat is used more efficiently, and therefore you don't seem to need as much. For myself, I have cut my food intake down to fifty percent of what it once was since doing these exercises every morning. The assimilation is so improved that hunger often disappears after doing the exercises with the body apparently absorbing available nutrients it would not have otherwise assimilated. And, as an average, I work a ten-hour day, with considerable demands on my physical strength and stamina. And, as mentioned elsewhere, I am almost sixty.

In staying young there is another important factor—retarding infection. The more we keep free of illness and infection, the healthier the interchange between blood and cellular tissue, which process in turn maintains and accelerates the rejuvenating process.

The lymphatic circulation, normally sluggish, has a great deal to do with our antibody production and resistance to disease. And this, of course, is improved with the exercises we advocate. The lymphatics appear to have the function of reducing pressure in the central nervous system, and this function is apparently initiated with exercise.

When I was in medical school, my anatomy professor told of a child he had examined who was crying continually, though there was apparently nothing wrong with him. The child had been ill, and had been in the crib for some days. The professor took the baby and gently bent its spine back and forth, with an accordion-like movement, and the baby almost immediately stopped crying. This movement had apparently been sufficient for the lymphatics to draw off excess spinal fluid and reduce the stress on the spinal cord. Later on, in pediatrics work, I remembered this technique in similar cases, where there seemed nothing wrong with an inactive child, and it worked. Through the years, with or without a scientific basis, I have learned to go ahead with anything that works. After all, it is the patient we are striving to help, not prove that one system of treatment is more advantageous than the other.

While all exercise, if not overdone, can be helpful in reconditioning the body, I prefer our gentle, subtle routines to the heavier calisthenics that the youthfully athletic favor in their gym work. As a young man, I have been through all this myself, lifting weights, chinning bars, climbing ropes, and swinging from parallel bars. However, these routines, designed to build muscular strength and prowess, have a different aim from ours. We are not after muscles. We are trying to develop endurance, vitality, longevity, good circulation, suppleness, flexibility, the ability to get in and out of tight corners, and primarily, yes, primarily, the peace of mind that goes along with confidence in our bodies to sustain us in moments of crisis. Our exercises are suited to the diminished muscular demands imposed on us as we go along in life. With women, of course, brute physical strength is seldom if ever desirable, and there is actually a reluctance to develop a muscular body which, while admirable in a young man, never looks well on a woman.

Actually, as we get older, with certain metabolic changes that occur around the ripe age of twenty-eight, it would be wiser to cut down gradually on the heavier types of physical exercise. At this stage of our lives, with the normal metabolic slowup, toxins often appear to build up faster under severe physical stress than the body can handily pass off. Even in their early thirties, wonderfully conditioned as they are, professional athletes, football, basketball, hockey, and even baseball players, who perform at a less arduous pace, complain of the pains and aches they have to work off.

Basically, beyond age thirty, weight-lifting or competitive sports with body contact, build up toxins that even an improved circulation can no longer carry off as readily as before. But we can stop worrying about this process if we do something relatively light to increase the circulation and limber the joints and muscles. The results are dramatically noticeable with exercises emphasizing stretching, breathing, relaxing, and joint motion.

In heavier exercise, the muscles are often limited in performance because of the stress placed on the joints. Frequently, in heavy work, tenderness develops in tendon attachments around knees, elbows and shoulders. We advocate not joint stress but joint motion increasing the flexibility of the joints.

Our exercises are slower, more rhythmic, associated with deep breathing. With this easy rhythmic approach we maintain an even interchange of oxygen and carbon dioxide so that the tissues don't accumulate large amounts of waste products, thereby increasing the efficiency of body movement, and discouraging fatigue.

It is gratifying to see how a healthy body will affect the individual's outlook, rekindling the optimism and humor that should be a constant companion through the viscissitudes of life.

Many patients have emotional problems that tend to make them nervous and diminish their self-confidence. These problems generally are aggravated in middle age, particularly if they deal with affairs of the heart. The individual is already concerned by the prospect of growing old, and his confidence in a sex relationship may be shaky at best—depending on his lady love's popularity, personality, and availability. I sometimes think of this as the middle-aged Lothario syndrome. And the lover is particularly vulnerable when the object of his affections is considerably younger than he, and there is a younger rival in the field.

One middle-aged Lothario had foolishly set his cap for a disinterested lady twenty years younger than he. And when he came in to see me, for a bad back, he had already received a "Dear John" letter. He was doubly inconsolable because of a displaced sacroiliac. Undoubtedly it had been helped out because of the emotional tension he was under. He was a sorry-looking individual. He couldn't eat or sleep, he couldn't work, his nerves were frayed. All he could talk about was getting away from it all.

"I think I'll get on the first plane for South America," he said.

His masculine ego had been wounded, and he wanted to be somewhere where he wouldn't be constantly reminded of his experience. He was like a cat on a hot tin roof. He couldn't sit still. And he wasn't thinking clearly. I told him as much.

"No matter where you go, you still have to take yourself with you. And you'd hardly be fun the way you are."

He glowered. "What do you suggest?"

"I suggest you should get yourself in shape."

"In shape for what?"

"For a younger and prettier girl."

I had caught his attention.

"And how do I do that?"

He was not in bad shape for his years, despite a middle-age paunch, jowls, and a mildly bloated look.

I gave him a list of Yoga-type exercises, and suggested he do them faithfully every day for two weeks. And then he was to come in again as I wanted to mark his progress.

I had appealed not only to his vanity, but to the instinct of self-preservation that we all have to a varying degree. He picked up the gauntlet I had thrown down. Two weeks later, when I next saw him, there was a new sparkle in his eye and a spring in his step. His waist was slimmer, the jowls had almost vanished, and the bloat was subdued. He had gone further than I had suggested, adopting a low-calorie vegetable diet. He looked years younger, and I enjoyed telling him as much.

With a smile, he told me he had booked a flight to Brazil. I nodded approval, for with his cheerful outlook and his spruced-up appearance he was certain to attract whatever it was he wanted.

"How about that girl?" I said. "Does she know you're leaving?"

He looked at me blankly. "What girl?" he said.

His recovery, I could see, was complete.

In the struggle to stay young, we generally equate slimness with youth. And the analogy is valid, as the human animal functions better in every respect without body fat. With our exercises there is a tendency for normalization, as the fat slim down and the thin fill out. But the main achievement is a feeling of well-being. After only a few weeks of exercise, patients have known what it is to feel energetic for the first time in years. Even when they tire toward the end of the day, they can snap out quickly with a shower or a bite to eat. They can freshen up by doing just a few minutes work, the Shoulder Stand,

and three or four exercises that relax the entire body and eliminate accumulated fatigue poisons.

We do not show age all at once. One of the first signs of aging is in the neck. The skin becomes raveled, and rather unsightly. However, the Head and Neck Roll helps keep this area firm, and the over-all exercises tend to have a tightening effect on the skin. These toning exercises, sending the blood into every cell, retard the loss of subcutaneous fat, which gives young women that rounded sensuous look, and masks ugly veins. This underlying fat is most prominently placed in the face, around the cheekbones, under the eyes, and in the body around the knees, elbows, and breastbone. When this is lost, the eyes frequently look sunken, and the knees and elbows get an unsightly bony look, with extra folds of loose skin.

Because of the aesthetic appeal of our exercises, I have been able to induce people, who would not ordinarily lift a finger, to inaugurate a daily routine of Yoga-type movements. At thirty-five, one patient was a sorry sight, tired and rundown, but he wouldn't hear of exercise until I mentioned the excellent results for people with receding hairlines.

He brushed a nervous hand through his own thinning locks, showing a bald spot as big as a silver dollar on the crown of his head.

"You mean I can get my hair back," he said incredulously.

"You may stop it falling out, and the color may come back."

What hair he had was a nondescript graying brown, reflecting his own lusterless self.

Many patients, after exercising, have a definite resurgence in hair growth, with a sharp rise in color. By increasing the circulation, and stimulating the glands and enzymes, the body makes better use of elements long dormant. Standing on the head definitely gives the hair follicles a fresh supply of blood. By feeding tissue with nutrients it requires, and has been recently lacking, you noticeably improve its function. This even applies to the teeth, as the same blood that helps the vision, hearing, and brain processes also nourishes and renews the gums, thus increasing the tone of the teeth. The teeth would decay without blood, as a blood vessel comes right to the tooth, and feeds it the required nutrients.

It is never too late to begin a reconditioning or rejuvenating program, and no background of physical training is required, though it is advised that you have a medical checkup first.

Offhand I cannot think of a worse physical specimen —ambulatory, that is—than the fifty-three-year-old housewife who presented herself as a back patient. Already, she had had a laminectomy, disc surgery, but her back was still stiff, paining excruciatingly when she bent over. She had leg pains, groin pains, shoulder pains. She had constant colds, a chronic stiffness of the neck, sinusitis. You name it and she had it, and if she didn't have it, she would get it. She had become a complainer on top of it all, and her mental attitude was one of "Woe is me." She was constantly tired, cranky, and pessimistic. If I had listened to her, I would have been depressed myself.

My first step, naturally, was to correct her sacroiliac, which, disc surgery or not, was severely displaced. It had been out of place for so long that she had considerable spasms in the lower back, which the surgery had done nothing for, and it was some time before we were able to relieve the pain in this area. Meanwhile, she complained of feeling cold, uncomfortable, short-breathed, fatigued, and unhappy. Some practitioners might have carted her off to the nearest psychiatrist. But I had seen patients like this before. As soon as her sacroiliac joint had stabilized, I felt a sound general exercise program was indicated. She looked at me as if I were out of my mind.

"At my age?" she said incredulously.

"Especially at your age," I said. "There's nothing wrong with you basically. Your heart is sound, your lungs are okay, and your digestion is adequate. You've just got to get some blood circulating through you again!"

When she continued to resist the idea of exercising, I suggested that she stop coming in as there was little more I could do for her. This seemed to make her realize I meant business.

"All right," she said, "what do I do?"

I gave her a list of exercises, such as the reader will find at the end of this book, and told her to proceed slowly, without strain. In the beginning, she was to just do two or three repetitions of the stretching and bending exercises, not bothering with the inverted exercises for a while, and gradually getting into more and more repetitions and more exercises as the weeks went by. She set her mind—and body—to it. The change was by no means dramatic, as there had been no sudden plunge into the routine. But she was a good pupil, and obediently followed the course I had laid out for her.

In a few weeks, she began to notice certain changes in herself. First and foremost, the general aches and pains disappeared, and she no longer felt cold and clammy all the time. There were even days when she woke up exhilarated, with her blood atingle. The increased circulation, as I suspected it would, was already affecting her blood flow and outlook on life, illustrating once more the direct effect of body chemistry on an individual's state of mind.

As her exercise routine broadened, she had ever more benefits to report. Amazingly, to her, she was no longer having trouble with her sinuses. The passages were no longer blocked, and the dull sinus ache had disappeared. While driving her car, she was now able to turn her neck without difficulty. There was more motion in her spine, as vertebrae calcium deposits broke down with improved circulation to these areas, induced through constant stretching and bending. Because of this stepped-up circulation, the chemistry around the joints was improved, and the tendons and ligaments agreeably affected. The synovial fluids, lubricating some joints, were once again active after a long, dry spell.

The change in the woman's attitude was well-nigh miraculous. Her husband and family were the principal beneficiaries, as they no longer had to listen to her complaints. But she was also beginning to enjoy life, taking pleasure now in preparing meals, a chore which she had previously transferred to the housekeeper. She enjoyed playing with her grandchildren, where they had been a burden before. She more than matched the agility of her daughter, who found herself wishing that she could do the things her mother was now capable of doing.

I had not seen her for months, when one day, out of the blue, I noticed her name in my appointment book. I sighed inwardly, thinking, What now? But I could have spared my misgivings. She arrived bright and cheerful, clad in a gay array of California colors, and looking ten years younger than when I had first seen her.

"I just wanted to show you what I can do," she said.

And then she proceeded to give me a demonstration. She bent forward, not only bringing her fingers to the floor but her palms. She bent backwards, so that her extended torso resembled the top of a table, and the supporting limbs the legs of that table. She cranked her head around a few times, expanded her chest and lungs, and even did the Shoulder Stand. It was a gratifying experience for her—and for me. Long after she left, I felt better for her demonstration. All of us need reassurance every now and then with the knowledge we are on the right track.

At any age, as long as you can manage motion, you can improve your body so it carries you instead of you carrying it. While I would not send an elderly person who has not exercised for years into a gym, I have not the same reserve about our rejuvenating routine because the movement is never strenuous and there is not the skeletal stress usually involved in exercises in the gym. We don't put a strain on the tissues and we move gradually into positions which require increased motion. All positions or postures start easily without stress, and are slowly moved ahead. You make a slight effort, but never pass the warning pain threshold. The means and the ends remain the same in our routine. Every day that we fully move a joint or a ligament that has not been moved in years we have made a signal advance.

CHAPTER X

More Rejuvenation

I am constantly impressed by the rejuvenation exercises, because that is precisely what they do. In rejuvenation, the health is directly benefited, and the improvement is generally dramatic, or we wouldn't use the superlative, *rejuvenate*. Somebody once said that when you are not unhappy, you are happy. By the same token, when you are not ill, you are healthy. As a doctor, I am inclined to equate rejuvenation with health, because that is what being young implies.

Different people, of course, age differently, and even if neither exercised, they might look ten or fifteen years different in age, and in the underlying condition that marks this discrepancy. For generally, after thirty, both as to physiognomy, facial characteristics, and body tone, the average person begins to look as he really is deep down inside.

Some people, accordingly, may respond more quickly and dramatically to the exercises, but all will respond, and in time even the laggard will equalize any discrepancies with the nonexerciser blessed with a youthful visage. The right exercise is a great equalizer. I have known men in their forties and fifties, who make a practice of physical fitness, who are not only dynamic in their business activities but who seem to transcend the age gap with the opposite sex, successfully courting young ladies many years their junior.

While I have no inclination to climb into the political arena, I can hardly ignore the accomplishments in a non-political text of United States Senator Strom Thurmond of South Carolina, who recently fathered two children. Though sixty-nine years of age, the senator is a tall, lean, powerfully built man, who looks no more than forty-five or fifty. As a physical fitness devotee, he practices some of the stretching and bending and flexing exercises we advocate, especially of an isometric nature, and it shows up not only in his physique but in his bearing, posture, and attitude toward life. His wife is only twenty-six, and though some might think this too great a disparity for a happy marriage, the marriage of this couple and their appearance together, belies this conventional belief.

It all begins in the mind. So imagine yourself as you want to be. Look into a mirror with your clothes off—if you can stand it—and picture yourself as you want to look to yourself, not to others. For this is a commitment that is preciously and privately your own. You are the most important person in the world to you. It all begins and ends with you. You can be no help to anybody—wife, husband, daughter, father, son, mother, or friend—unless you have worked out your own problems, and your health and approach to life is at the nub of these problems.

No person who is ill all the time, regardless of age, is

youthful. You know how tiresome people like this can be, with their constant complaints and excuses, so do everything you can not to be one of them.

Once you begin the exercises you have already made a decision that will have far-reaching impact on your health. The decision itself is a big step forward, the exercises themselves are the follow through. On innumerable occasions I have seen good health flow out of this simple decision that people have made to do something about themselves—to retard the aging processes which would relegate them to the human junk heap long before they are emotionally ready for it. Indeed, the people who do these exercises conscientiously never reach this stage—they are productive about themselves, and thus become productive in everything they turn their hand to.

They cannot afford to be ill, not even for a day. They cannot afford pesky colds, chilblains, incapacitating headaches, lumbar backaches, sinus problems, and the veritable array of maladies that unresisting man is heir to. I regularly note the beneficial impact of our exercises on everyday health patterns. The common cold is debilitating and a nuisance, and I have treated it effectively with large doses of natural vitamin C. However, patients with upper respiratory infections have frequently aborted them with the exercises we recommend. When you start to sniffle, go into the Shoulder Stand and stay four or five minutes, if you can do it comfortably. When you try this posture again, two or three hours later, your nose is freer, your throat doesn't rasp as much, and the malaise accompanying these symptoms is gone. Doing the exercises routinely, you will find that the initial cold symptoms often disappear in a few hours, provided that you don't work against your strength.

Patients, once subject to colds, will go for years, or forever, without again suffering this nuisance. Heightened circulation improves the resistance, and new confidence in one's ability to mobilize his body may also inspire a newfound immunity. More and more we realize the great influence of mind on body.

But even where suggestibility is negligible, striking results emerge from these exercises. A fifty-year-old patient, in otherwise good shape, reported a loss of hearing with some consternation. For months he had thought that people were mumbling to him. And then one day, when the telephone rang in the next room, and everyone heard it clearly but him, he realized his hearing was off. He associated his hearing loss with a whiplash injury he had suffered a year before, convincing himself that his feeling that people were mumbling started at that time. Accordingly, he consulted a prominent ear specialist in Beverly Hills. After an intensive examination, the specialist reported that the patient had lost thirty-five percent of his hearing in both ears. He blamed a degenerative nerve process common in some families after forty.

"Could an automobile accident have touched it off?" the patient inquired, thinking of possible remedies.

The specialist shook his head. "Not a chance."

Our patient, a well-known publicist, thought a moment. "What can I do about it?" he asked.

The doctor shrugged. "Come back in a year and I'll fit you for a hearing aid."

The deterioration was of a hereditary nature, and always, the specialist said, ended in deafness or near-deafness.

The patient remembered now that his mother, brother, and others in his family had suffered a severe hearing loss after forty, but saw some hope for himself since his hearing had continued to be excellent long beyond that age. He still felt it had something to do with the accident.

He came to me thinking that perhaps an impinged nerve had affected his hearing, and that a spinal adjustment, relieving pressure points, might bring his hearing back. I was sorry that I had to disabuse him. Checking him over, I saw that he was a fine physical specimen. He was in tiptop condition, with good body tone, splendid musculature, and a flat stomach. There was not a vertebra out of place, and his spine was strong and flexible. I told him he showed no significant effects from his automobile accident.

My diagnosis was similar to the specialist's. As some people get older, the ossicles of the inner ear often harden, atrophying nerves essential to the conduction of sound. And this condition, though of a hereditary nature, usually occurs when the tissues form calcium deposits at a time of life when the flow of blood to the head has noticeably decreased.

But since he did Yoga exercises which bring blood to the head, I was surprised that his hearing had been affected.

"Standing on your head or doing the Shoulder Stand should have reduced the deposits," I pointed out.

My patient looked up sharply. "But I haven't done these exercises since my accident. The man who treated me said the Shoulder Stand or the Headstand would only aggravate my whiplash."

"Go back to the Headstand and the Shoulder Stand," I told him, "and do each for five minutes or as long as you are comfortable."

The results were gratifying. In three weeks, he noted a hearing improvement, and in five weeks, he could clearly hear the telephone in the next room. In three months, he could hear the tick of his watch on his night table, a sound he hadn't heard for almost a year.

Generally speaking, I find people in their forties and fifties much more concerned than the younger people with maintaining their youthful vigor and health. I suppose it is axiomatic that we never really appreciate anything until we are in danger of losing it. However, younger people have just as much need of these exercises, as they constantly overextend themselves in the blind confidence of youth. While the older group is more co-operative, many young people become tractable when the only alternative is excruciating pain.

A twenty-year-old ski instructor came in with low-back pain, which made it difficult for him to do the skiing turns he was teaching. I showed him the corrective exercise after adjusting his sacroiliac, and then discussed the conditioning exercises. He replied that he was getting enough exercise on the snow slopes and fighting forest fires—his avocation. I pointed out that our exercises specifically prepared the ligaments for the special stress of skiing. By stretching your tissues every day in a regular routine, I told him, you minimize the possibilities of overstretching on skis. It made sense to him, and I outlined the exercises.

He spends twenty or twenty-five minutes a day at them now, and reports that he has more vitality than ever, is much more flexible, and even skis better. His back problem has disappeared.

I urge that the exercises be done every day. Otherwise, as we pass thirty-five or forty, they become more difficult after only a two-day layoff. The fibrous tissues that surround the joints tighten up after twenty-four hours or so of being idle. It becomes harder to stretch, and some elasticity is lost. We can start at any age, with the slightest motion, the important thing is following through with at least a little every day. Begin gradually, with only the movement of a hand, if that is all you can do. If a joint in the finger is stiff, move it a little more each day, until there is normal motion. The same applies to every joint in the body. In days, weeks, months, progress will be noticeable and lasting. By just making an effort, you re-educate the nerve stimulus, and it becomes stronger daily, until nerve and joint are once more meshed together co-operatively.

Even in a wheelchair, if the heart is unaffected, it is possible to make a start. The very thought of moving a finger previously immovable is a help. As you keep thinking about moving that finger or joint, wrist or elbow, little by little you increase function in that area. The mind puts out the first stimulus, and movement results. So just thinking about it, concentrating hard on it, is all-important. In developing this concentration, you have an extra bonus, for this same concentration can be applied to every function in time, giving you total control of yourself.

Anybody can do *some* of these exercises. The average

person, who hasn't been active, should be able to undertake a routine embracing about half of the exercises. There is no need for people who see the diagrams and pictures of these exercises to immediately reproduce these positions. The exercises are to be done gradually, slowly and over a period of time. They can be fully achieved in one, two, three, four, or five years, depending on the individual's age, physical condition, and requirements. As you continue the exercises, you will find that they become easier and more rewarding. And the improvement in the way you function, not only on the exercise mat, but in just moving about casually will become noticeable to you and others.

The first result, surprisingly, will be one of inward relaxation. You will start to relax mentally and emotionally within two or three weeks, even before you have noticed any real physical change. As you gain more control of your body and of your mind through concentration, you will find that you sleep and rest better. Some patients with insomnia problems have reported that after a few weeks of the exercises, they are able to drop off to sleep in the daytime, in resuscitating naps, for the first time in their lives.

Moderation in all things, including our exercises, is the keynote. The exercises are to be done without strain, particularly in the beginning. Even the corrective exercise is to be done gently, without pushing yourself or your muscles. As you do each exercise, the body will begin to gradually expand and slowly stretch the tissues so that they adapt very naturally. As you go along, your strengthened tissues will call on you to increase the repetitions of each exercise, as your endurance is increased almost without your realizing it. Where you started with two or three motions or repetitions the first time, in a few weeks you will easily be doing the ten repetitions that I consider sufficient for any single exercise. Your own increased flexibility will surprise you in time, so long as you proceed patiently, and think only in terms of your own improvement, not what somebody else can do. Increased motion and endurance is the barometer of your progress. There is no age limit. If an individual can do anything at all, flex his legs, raise or lower his arms, or move any part of his body in any direction at all, he is eligible for improvement and a bold, brave, new life, in which he becomes the master of not only body but mind.

He can start at age four or five, or eighty or ninety, just so, as I noted before, that he can send an impulse from his brain to his finger. Where the person is not very flexible, I would defer the Shoulder Stand and the Headstand —doing the Plough and the leg elevations to strengthen the lower back so that he can eventually get up in the Shoulder Stand. Also, it is a good idea to slowly and gradually bring about the increased circulation to the head, as a drastic circulatory change, such as the Shoulder Stand or the Headstand produces, might make one dizzy or cause him to blackout in the beginning.

Remember, at all times, that the exercises should be done slowly and in rhythm with deep breathing. Never concentrate on any exercise to a point where you forget the breathing and hold your breath. The breathing is vital, and becomes as much a part of the exercise as the movement of joint, muscle, and ligament.

It is advisable to choose one set hour of day for the exercises, since we are all creatures of habit and our bodies become receptive to the exercises at their accustomed time. I prefer my routine before breakfast, but other people find it convenient to relax with the exercises after their workday, just before dinner, or before going to bed, when the easy rhythm may prepare you for restful slumber. The exercises should never be done directly after eating, particularly the inverted exercises. They should be done a minimum of three hours after a meal and preferably four hours. That is why I suggest the morning routine after rising.

However, you are stiffer in the morning, and the exercises are more difficult then, because you haven't moved your joints or ligaments for seven or eight hours, though the body does toss about twenty-five or thirty times during a night of slumber, without stimulating circulation or flexibility. In the morning, the circulation is still sluggish, and the tissues are not as adaptable as they will be after two or three hours of normal activity. Even experienced Yogis put off the Headstand or Shoulder Stand for hours after rising, as there is a tendency for the muscles in the shoulders and neck, still stiff in the morning, to cramp or form spasms in these inverted postures at this time.

Later in the day, the same movement is effortless and the reaction is a pleasant one. When your blood is being forced into the tissues, it results in relaxed tissue action. If the blood flow is cut way down for even a short time, then this relaxing action ceases, and stiffening ensues.

As you continue to do these exercises, you may note the diminution of facial lines and wrinkles caused by a loss of

that subcutaneous fat which gives an impression of round-
ness and firmness. We don't get any of this soft tissue
back, but as we do our exercises we improve muscle tone
to the point of tightening the skin. In expanding underlying muscle tissues, less looseness in the skin obviously results.

The ailing can be helped too. Some patients have a
chronic inflammation of the ligaments of the vertebrae. It
is a fairly common condition, limiting the motion of the
spine to a point where the person can hardly move his spinal column. By increasing circulation to the ligaments, via
the spinal lift or Cobra exercise, we bring blood to these
ligaments, increasing the elimination of toxins which are a
byproduct of metabolism. When we can do this with an
ailing spine, we can do so much more with a spine whose
only problem is a functional stiffening with time and age.
Somebody once said that you are as young as your spine.
As the center of the nervous system, the spine influences
every body function for better or worse. So bear in mind
at all times the importance of increasing spinal motion and
flexibility in our exercises.

The exercises should be performed in a relaxed atmosphere, as comfortably as possible. You should be dressed
comfortably and loosely in nonbinding clothes, free of
belts or sashes and shoes, yet warm enough to hold in the
body heat and not allow the muscles to chill during rest
periods. I advise leotards for the ladies, and sweatsuits for
both men and women, as they are not only warm and
roomy, but convey the feeling that you are well equipped
for the exercises you are about to do.

The room should be light and airy, with the temperature ranging between 68 and 72 degrees. Though it is fine to keep windows open, there should be no drafts. Air should circulate indirectly, so that when you become warm or perspire, you will avoid a severe muscular reaction. The floor should be covered with carpeting, and a body-length exercise mat laid down over the rug. When lying down, there should be no pressure on the pubic bones, buttocks, shoulders, neck, knees, or head.

Before each routine get in a relaxed state of mind. Visualize each exercise, indeed each movement in each exercise, getting it well fixed in the mind. In the beginning, rest comfortably between the exercises, sitting with the legs crossed if you like, resting for as long as you took for the last exercise. Visualization is valuable because in imagining the exercises you imagine them perfectly, and so set up the subconscious patterns for doing them perfectly. In time, you will do as well as you imagine.

As proper breathing is so vital to all the exercises, as it is in all of life, take several deep breaths between each exercise, as well as being very conscious of your breathing during the exercises themselves. Actually your first exercise should be diaphragmatic breathing to load the system with oxygen, and lessen the likelihood of fatigue.

Many of these Yoga-style exercises are modified in such a way as to give added stress in areas where I feel it especially needed for maximum flexibility and glandular impact with an economy of effort. Western man has different needs than his Eastern brother. He requires more activation and stimulation to better participate in the tide of events swirling about him. He needs energy and enterprise as well as peace of mind, and in the fullest exploitation of these energies he often finds the inner peace that has escaped him.

Do not be disturbed if you cannot do very much at first. Please remember in all these exercises that the attainment of the exercise or posture is not as important as the concentration and effort that goes into attempting the exercise. The ends and the means are the same in our Yoga-style routine, just as they are in life. So do only your best, and the best will come back to you.

CHAPTER XI

Our Rejuvenation Exercises

DEEP BREATHING

With the breath we take, we replenish body, mind, and spirit. The old Yogis spoke of the breath of life, the pranyama, and with this breath we take from the substance of the universe around us and gather strength from this substance with our vitalic breathing. We breathe with every cell of our body, visualizing the new life that is being sent through us with every breath we take. We breathe to live and live to breathe. It is a harmonious cycle, which we must never forgo as we do our exercises— and, just as importantly, carry on into other activities.

Breathing is always the first exercise, and an important part of every other exercise. You can breathe sitting, standing, or lying down. However, I have found that many people find it easier to visualize the breathing exercise in a squatting or sitting position. So, as a starter, if your muscles and joints permit, just sit on the floor in a semi-lotus position if possible. It doesn't have to be perfect, or near-perfect. Just squat in as comfortable a position as you can get in, on the floor or mat, with your legs lightly crossed at the ankles, and your hands resting easily in your lap, palms up. Visualize your diaphragm, and your lungs, think of the oxygen streaming through your blood, and feeding every cell and tissue in your body—your heart, lungs, brain, liver, pancreas, kidneys, every organ and every cell. As you think this, you can express this thought to yourself or even aloud. It will serve to reinforce the picture you have drawn of the help you are getting. Now in this relaxed state of mind and body, take a deep breath through your nose and blow it out forcefully through the mouth to clear your lungs quickly of any stale air that may be there.

In the next step, inhaling through the nose as usual, we breathe deeply, striving for the count of ten with one breath retention, and exhaling to a similar ten count. If you cannot do this in the beginning, start with any count that you can comfortably take a single breath to, whether it's two, three, four or five. But remember you cannot harm yourself breathing in at ten, or exhaling to that count. Eventually, you will work up to twenty-five and thirty seconds, if you wish, but for a starter, ten will be sufficient. In inhaling, let the stomach relax and balloon out. Exhaling, pull stomach in. The diaphragm contracts and rises during exhalations, relaxes and falls during inhalations, helping the air to reach the lower lung where it is widest and most capacious. It is important to fully expel the stale air. There is no point to absorbing great bursts of air if all one does is push the stale air deeper down into the lung pockets. In emptying the lungs thoroughly, fresh air will then rush in automatically as nature abhors a vacuum.

There are a few aids to doing the breathing exercise properly. In sitting erect, with the legs folded crosswise, place one hand on the stomach, and the other on the chest. While inhaling, allow the lower hand to move out with the stomach as it balloons out. Exhaling, lower hand should move in, as the stomach contracts. The hand on the chest should not move at all, as there should be no heaving of the shoulders or chest. The back must be straight, and you should try to isolate the muscles of the abdominal area, and move only them.

Deep breathing has a generally calming effect on the whole personality, reducing jumpiness and nervous tension. The creatures that breathe more rapidly than man tend to be more restless and short-lived. Monkeys have almost twice man's respiration rate, whereas the long-lived elephant and tortoise are slow breathers. Curiously, children and primitive peoples, as well as animals, use their diaphragms more than adult people in their normal breathing, noticeably relaxing their abdomens. As you concentrate on your breathing, developing an easy rhythm, you will learn to control it automatically, and it will become slower and easier. After a while, under stress, or crisis, you may be able to deliberately slow your breathing to a point where nervousness predictably decreases and composure is induced.

You may prefer to do your diaphragmatic breathing standing, which is all right, so long as you are more comfortable this way. The procedure doesn't vary much from what it is in the semi-lotus posture. And whatever applies to the standing-breathing exercise applies also to the sitting position, and vice versa. In practicing these exercises, progress should be soon noted in increased oxygen flow, improved mental concentration, new breath control, isolation of muscle movement, and the ability to visualize—all together serving to fully develop your subconscious potential.

The breathing in these exercises cannot be overemphasized. Standing, breathe in deeply five or six times, forcing the air right down to the diaphragm, and then send it up and out by contracting the abdominal muscles. You will feel increased warmth and energy, as the bottom of your lungs is at last introduced to life-giving oxygen. You may eventually work up to breathing in and out rapidly fifty or sixty times, inhaling and exhaling through the nose, your speed increasing as you manage through practice to contract the diaphragm area both swiftly and rhythmically. Some, as they learn to contract and expand the abdomen in staccato fashion, have lost as much as two inches around the waist from this exercise alone.

Diaphragmatic breathing can also be done lying down. The hands again are placed on the stomach and chest to check that the breathing is being done properly, with only the abdominal muscles contracting and expanding to force the air down and out of the lungs. Ideally, you should expand the lungs in stages, first the lower, then the middle area, and finally the top of the lungs, as one would fill a cup. Although it is well to concentrate on the breathing in the beginning, after a while it will become second nature and you can breathe automatically, without even thinking about it.

As simple as it is, deep diaphragmatic breathing has relieved asthma, emphysema, and other respiratory problems, including shortness of breath. In asthma clinics, in treating a child, therapists will place a toy duck on a child's stomach and ask the child to make the duck rise and fall as though it were sitting on rolling waves.

Visualization during breathing cannot be overstressed. As an aid in relieving nervousness, visualize with each breath a calm blue sea with waves slowly rising and falling to the rhythm of the breathing.

Visualization is as important in this breathing exercise as in any other movement, and breathing properly is definitely a movement. For additional benefits you may vary the diaphragmatic breathing, as you progress with this breathing exercise. Twist your body about in a half circle, as you proceed to breathe in, expanding the diaphragm, and contract the diaphragm quickly as you breathe out.

In this exercise, standing up in a twisted position, you are at approximately a 45-degree rotation when you take your first deep breath, pushing out the diaphragm or abdomen as you do. As you breathe, visualize the diaphragm moving up and down rhythmically. And then think of the torso being turned in such a way from the hips so that all of the organs in the abdomen are moving up and down in unison with the diaphragm. Consider that you are pushing your liver up and down, your kidneys, your spleen, pancreas, and even the stomach. Only in this position, in this torso twist, are these organs actually being pressed down in such a way that they are getting a veritable internal massage with a healthful renewal of circulation.

After breathing in and out in this position for five or six times, building up repetitions gradually, twist the trunk in the other direction, reversing it 180 degrees, to take a completely opposite position. Repeat the exercise, inhaling and exhaling rhythmically with each diaphragmatic movement, massaging these organs in just the opposite position they were before.

There is no more invigorating exercise than diaphragmatic breathing with the trunk turned. You are not only getting the muscular benefits from the twist under the subtle tension of deep breathing, but by increasing the internal circulation you improve the tone of tissue which ordinarily does not receive any beneficial stimulation. Your visceral organs should maintain the same even tone that your muscles do. Increased circulation in this area makes the secretory mechanisms more efficient, and is a vital factor in assuring long life and youthfulness. Ordinary calisthenics, contrarily, do not directly stimulate the abdominal or visceral organs, nor make deep breathing an essential part of their exercise program.

Normally, people are low on oxygen. The necessary interchange between the oxygen inflow, and the carbon dioxide expelled is often impeded by the fact that people ordinarily do not breathe deeply enough to eliminate the carbon dioxide waste which is a byproduct of body metabolism. Many people just breathe in their chests. Their ribs expand, and they get air to the top of their lungs, and the middle, if lucky. Rarely does it get to the bottom, and force out the stale toxic air which is there.

Sooner or later, all this trouble to breathe properly will reap its own reward. After a while, you will notice in taking a long walk, gardening, climbing a hill, that you are breathing deeply and easily, without thinking about it and your endurance is greater than it has been for years. Subconsciously, the new breathing pattern has become a habit, with the capacity for doing things consequently increased.

We have spent all this time with these breathing exercises, because oxygen is the body's most vital fuel. Learn how to use it, not lose it. Plant the thought that you will breathe properly at all times, in deeply with each upward movement of the body and limbs, out deeply with each downward movement. In time, the breathing will become as much a part of the exercise as the body movements. Your subconscious mind is being programed to perform naturally and properly at all times.

After the breathing stint, turn to a simple stretching exercise that all of you should be able to do handily.

SPINE STRETCH

The Spine Stretch is the first movement in our routine. Lie down comfortably on your back on the floor, extending both arms over the head as far behind you as you can with your legs extended, toes pointed, trying to get in the last full stretch. Breathing in as arms and legs go out, breathing out as you relax them, return the arms to their original position, palms down at hips. Stretch the right arm over head and extend the right leg as far as possible, pressing the trunk firmly to the floor. Now relax the right arm and the right leg, allowing them to rest, and breathe in deeply. Relax and breathe out as you bring arm to original position. Repeat with the left arm and left leg. Stretch the right arm and left leg, breathing in. Breathing out return the right arm and the left leg. Now breathing in, stretch the left arm and the right leg. Return to original position and breathe out. Relax and take a few deep breaths. You have finished your spine stretching exercise.

This exercise, with its various movements, is done just once. Its purpose is simple. It limbers slumbering muscles and joints, and allows you to get in the habit of breathing properly while doing the exercises. As a rule, we breathe in through the nose with any upward movement of the arms, torso, legs or neck, and exhale through the nose or mouth as we bend forward, or lower our arms, leg, or head. Stretching stimulates the circulation in a very gentle way and contributes to the elasticity of ligaments, tendons, and joints. The farther you stretch, gradually there is less likelihood of injury at work or play by a sudden awkward movement. Your radius of movement will become wider to accommodate any workaday demand the body puts on it.

Let me again stress the breathing, repeating perhaps what I have already said, and throwing in a few new pointers. As every movement is instigated, the deep-breathing process begins. As you stretch one particular area of your body, breathe in deeply. As you relax the motion, let the air out, trying to cultivate an easy rhythm between the movement and the breathing, as if making them one. Although it is permissible to exhale through the mouth, it is preferable to breathe in and out through the nose, as long as there is no nasal obstruction. Breathing out through the nose clears the dust and particles trapped by the fine, silky hairs in the nose. It also warms the air as it comes into the bronchial passages and the lungs, and helps establish an easy and productive rhythm.

Oxygen is more important than food and water in fueling the body and making it work. We can do without food for several weeks, water a day or two as a rule, but oxygen, generally no more than two or three minutes. Our goal is to get enough oxygen into our lungs to enrich our blood, oxygenate our system, and make the human machine function smoother and easier. You will find in the beginning that as you breathe in and out consciously with each movement that the exercises become simpler to do. If you experiment, breathing as you do normally, without a conscious effort at deep breathing, you will find the same exercise far more difficult, with considerably more energy required to do the same number of repetitions.

ROCK 'N ROLL

The Rock 'N Roll is also known as the Supine Roll. Sit upright on the floor, cross the ankles, with knees in upright position, and leaning forward, firmly grasp the opposite toes with each hand. Still flexing forward, bring the head toward the knees, and form an arch or semicircle with the spine. You are now ready, holding on to your toes and taking a simultaneous deep breath, to roll back on your spine. Your crossed feet come back over your head, which is now resting on the floor, and almost touch the floor if possible. Expelling the breath forcefully, rock forward a bit, and giving the head a forward thrust, roll up to a full sitting position. Start with two or three rolls, then gradually increase to ten. Uniquely, breathe in as you roll back, and out as you come forward, the intake of breath and the exhalation helping to provide the momentum required to start the roll backwards and forwards. As you perform this exercise, visualize the spine and each vertebra separately as it contacts the floor, one ridge at a time, as you would visualize a barrel and its separate staves. This exercise tends not only to increase the flexibility of the spine, but may move a vertebra back in place if it is out, or release locked muscles which have been in spasm.

THE PLOUGH

Lie flat on your back on the floor with the hands forward, palms down at the hips. Raise both legs together slowly, while inhaling, keeping palms pressed down on the floor. Without bending knees, and with your toes pointed, continue to raise hips and back, bringing the legs up over the head, with the knees still straight, and exhaling as the toes reach for the floor behind. Breathe slowly in and out through the nose, tucking the chin into the thyroid notch of the throat. As a variation of the Plough, swing the arms back from in front of you and grasp the toes, providing an extra stretch. In the beginning, if you cannot reach the floor with your toes, do not be discouraged. You will, and sooner than you think. Go as far as you can, and hold the position in a relaxed way, taking deep breaths. Hold position for two or three breaths in the beginning, eventually advancing to ten breaths. Then with arms extended in front of you, palms pressed down to the floor, and breathing out, bring legs slowly back to the floor to a horizontal position. You increase the flexibility of the spine, and send fresh blood to the head, neck, and throat. You stimulate the glands in the throat with this added circulation, and the thyroid by the chin's pressure to the throat. Because of thyroid stimulation, many consider this a sex exercise. Be that as it may, the increased circulation benefits organs in the head, scalp, and upper body. The large muscles back of the thighs are stretched, and congestion in the legs reduced. With the lymph and blood draining from the legs, a tendency toward varicose veins may be diminished, as long as you do the exercise. The thyroid gland is generally in a state of imbalance, and this exercise tends to normalize this delicate butterfly-shaped gland. Normalization of this gland may also produce a more complete metabolism, and touch off a chain reaction improving the performance of the entire endocrine system. A person with a hyperactive thyroid will relax with this exercise and be less irritable. It may also slow down rapid beating of the heart and eliminate the tremors common with this hyperactivity.

THE LOCUST

As a rule, if we arch the back one way in an exercise, we bend in the opposite direction next to maintain an even flexibility. In the Locust, you lie on the floor face down, arms drawn back at the sides with the fists closed and the thumbs down or with the hands under the groin, palms up. Keep the legs straight. Inhale deeply as you elevate the feet and legs, keeping the knees stiff, so as to arch the spine while keeping the chest on the floor. Maintain this position with your legs ideally vertical. However, in the beginning, just getting the feet off the floor will be satisfactory. Hold for five to fifteen seconds. Then, slowly let the legs down, breathing out with this movement. Repeat this exercise two or three times as a starter, eventually building up to ten repetitions. There should be no bending at the knee, the straightness of the legs helping to form the arch in the spine. Your clenched hands down on the floor provide a lever for the leg raise. Reversing the stress of the Plough, the Locust increases the mobility of the spine, stretching the anterior spinal ligaments. It also tightens the muscles of the lower back, abdomen, thighs, and the buttocks. Increased stimulation to the pelvic area benefits the glands in this area, the fresh circulation to the uterus or prostate gland improving their tone and function.

THE SHOULDER STAND

The Shoulder Stand is sometimes called the Good-for-Everything exercise. It is an inverted exercise usually done handily before the Headstand is even attempted. The Shoulder Stand is done in a vertical position with the shoulders and back of neck resting comfortably on the floor. The legs are extended straight above the body, the back arched, the buttocks pulled in, and the chin tucked into the notch of the throat, stimulating thyroid circulation. The hands fall back to the small of the back to support the vertical posture, but in time you will rest comfortably on your shoulders and cervicals without this support.

To derive top benefit from this position, lie flat on the back, arms extended at side, palms down at hips. As you inhale, elevate the legs, with the knees bent, arching the back until the trunk attains a vertical position, with elbows on the floor and hands supporting the small of the back. Extend legs straight up from the hips, with the toes pointed to the ceiling. You should be able to drop a plumbline from toe to shoulder. Stay as straight as possible, keeping the feet from waving back and forth. Don't forget to breathe in and out. There is a tendency for the novice to hold his breath as he concentrates on a holding posture. This exercise improves circulation to the scalp, eyes, ears, throat, sinuses. In reversing the normal pull of gravity, it helps sagging organs in the abdominal tract to resume original positions. With women, a retroverted uterus may assume a natural pelvic position because of reverse gravity. Similarly, pressure on tubes from the kidney to the bladder may be eased. Spleen, pancreas, and liver all rest comfortably in this inverted position, and gain a new circulatory response which is stimulating and beneficial for the organs, as well as muscles, ligaments, and tendons. Drainage from the sinuses, bronchial tubes, lungs is notably improved.

Stay up as long as you can, striving gradually to maintain this posture for three minutes. In coming out of this position, bend the knees first, then extend hands to side, palms down. Lower your legs gradually, releasing chin from throat on way down and flattening back against the floor. Maintain disciplined movement in regaining a re-laxed position, not allowing legs to dangle.

Do this exercise only once.

With increased flow of blood to the upper body, throat and head, an increased resistance to infection develops in these areas, as the aroused lymphatics stimulate germ-fighting antibodies. This exercise can be done safely as long as you are not fatigued by your illness and there is no fever.

In the Shoulder Stand, as the Headstand, the results are multiple. There is a certain aesthetic or cosmetic benefit, with the blood renewing the tired facial tissue, and bringing back that fresh glow of long ago. Immediately after the Shoulder Stand, with the blood still suffusing the facial area, rub the face vigorously for a few seconds to bring the blood tingling to the skin.

Elsewhere, we have mentioned the benefit of the Headstand in degenerative deafness. The Shoulder Stand, too, can claim credit in this connection. By increasing the blood flow to the semicircular canals, the hearing may be dramatically improved. Where catarrhal deafness is a factor, clogging the eustacian tubes, the hearing may be notably improved as congestion is relieved. In some instances, a fifty percent hearing loss may be restored to normal. The restoration may occur over a period of a few days, or a few weeks, depending on your persistence and the seriousness of the catarrhal problem.

Again, as with the Headstand, there is a tremendous increase in hair health, and hair may grow where there was a hair loss before.

For the elderly, with waning circulation to the extremities, I particularly recommend this exercise, so long as they start slowly. In the beginning, I suggest just a momentary position until the oldsters gain enough strength and flexibility from the supine exercises to be able to gradually arch their backs and rest comfortably on their shoulders. The increased circulation, where there has been little circulation before, seems to increase the alertness of the individual and help maintain memory patterns in relationship to the present. Some in their seventies have been able to maintain the Shoulder Stand for three of four minutes with ease. And what a few can do, others can strive for.

THE COBRA

Lie on the stomach, fully stretched out, with palms pressing against the floor at shoulder level, the fingers forward or inclined toward each other. As you breathe in, lift the head in a snakelike motion, then successively raise neck, shoulders, and lower back, raising the spine as far as possible, while keeping the lower body flat on the floor from the hips down. Lift slowly, and try to feel the snake-like uncoiling of the spine vertebra by vertebra. Push up from the arms as the shoulders and head rise vertically, or as far as possible at the peak of the exercise. Breathe in slowly coming up, and out in the same rhythm going down, synchronizing with a ten count both up and down. At the summit, hold for a few moments, and stretch from the hips up, neck, shoulders, and spine. Now from the hips, lower your body as slowly as you raised it, until the head touches the floor. Do this exercise two or three times to begin with, and gradually work up to ten repetitions. There is no more relaxing exercise. It is a specific for the back. You increase circulation and motion in the spine, benefiting nerves, muscle, and tissue relating to the spinal column. The neck and shoulders also benefit from the improved stretch, and the muscles in forearms and wrists are strengthened appreciably.

ALL FOURS

After finishing the Cobra, relax on back for a few moments, taking a couple of deep breaths, and then crawl around on hands and knees for ten or fifteen seconds for a change of pace. As your back gets more supple, you can vary this by humping your back and walking stiff-legged on your hands and feet in a sort of bear walk. It's invigorating fun, and you should enjoy these exercises.

THE BODY TWIST

The Body Twist is a relatively easy exercise to do, but a hard one to describe. Veritably, a descriptive illustration or picture is worth a thousand words, but we shall try to describe this exercise so that you will be sure to profit from the unique stresses it puts on your system.

Sit with legs extended, palms down beside the knees. Take a deep breath and fold the right leg at the knee and then breathing out cross right leg over the left leg in the sitting position. Then bring the left heel up to the buttocks on the right side, meanwhile breathing rhythmically with each movement. You should now be sitting straight up, your right knee and right thigh are close to your chest, your right foot is outside the left knee which is flat on the floor, and the left foot is on its side with the heel next to the right buttock. To accomplish the Body Twist, now bring the left arm along the outer side of the upraised right knee and try to grasp toes of left foot. Then, with the trunk vertical, though twisted, bring the right arm around the back and hold at waist level.

At the same time, turn head and look around as far as possible over the right shoulder so that the twist is felt all the way up the spine and neck. Repeat this exercise crossing the left leg over the right, and repeating the movements on this side in reverse, remembering to breathe in and out.

As you hold the Body Twist position, take a diaphragmatic breath to the count of ten, or whatever you can comfortably, and then let out the breath to a similar count slowly and easily. Deep breathing at this time, because of the turn of the torso, serves to stimulate through the gentle pressure of internal massage the circulation into the vital organs—the liver, kidneys, spleen, pancreas—and should improve their tone. The breathing may be repeated two or three times on one side, and then done again when the Body Twist is performed on the reverse side. The pelvic region is firmly anchored during this variation of the twist, providing a lateral stretch far more beneficial than undisciplined hip-swinging. The lungs are expanded and more flexible, and the internal massage often relieves congestion in the viscera. Stretched upper and lower vertebrae become more elastic. Study this exercise, and do it. It is good for you.

HEAD-TO-KNEE POSTURE

Here is another great body stretcher. The movement stretches the muscles back of the legs and the lower spine, and brings a needed flexibility to the pelvic bones or hipbones, so important in resisting sacroiliac problems. It also conditions the recreative organs and is good for what ails most of us after forty. It is a simple exercise, not hard to master.

Take a couple of deep breaths, then sit up and extend your legs till the feet are about three feet apart. Take the right heel and fold it into the groin, against the pubic bones, the sole of the foot pressed against the thigh if possible. If you can't bring the heel in all the way, bring it in as far possible, with the knee flat to the floor or as close to it as you can manage. Gently press knee to floor and feel the hip joint relax. Raise arms high over head, inhaling. Then reach forward, breathing out, and bring hands to the extended ankle or, if possible, catch the toes. Almost in a follow-through motion, gradually lower head and forehead to the extended knee, holding this posture for a few seconds if you can. Then raise the arms and breathe in as you resume original sitting position. Repeat this exercise with the other leg extended, inhaling again as you raise arms high over the head, remembering to breathe out as head is lowered to the opposite knee. Repeat this exercise on both sides three times, then relax, and take a few deep breaths. You are now in the middle of the workout, and should be warmed up. Guard against fatigue, and do not overdo. Rest between exercises. Do not proceed to the next exercise if you are even slightly winded or your heartbeat is faster than normal.

NECK ROLLS

The Neck Rolls can be done standing, sitting, even lying down, if you prefer. Some find the sitting position most comfortable, with the legs crossed in front. To begin, turn your head as far to the left as you can without strain, breathing in. Then bring your head back to the starting position, and turn the head to the right. Repeat three times in each direction to prepare for the roll itself. Flex your chin down as far as you can on the chest. Then bring the head back over your shoulders. Repeat this movement—down and back—three times, gently and easily, taking a deep breath as the head goes back, and breathing out as it comes forward. Lifting neck, slowly rotate head from center all the way around, dropping it towards the shoulders in back, and on the chest up front, taking a count of fifteen or twenty to complete each rotation. Repeat the roll three times in each direction, remembering to breathe in and out.

Do not turn just the face, but make sure the head is revolving, lolling on chest and shoulders as it revolves. If you hear a gritty noise, it only means you need this exercise to loosen calcium deposits in the cervical vertebrae. The rolls relax the neck muscles and a cervical area so often taut with the stress of the day. Increasing circulation to the neck, the rolls stimulate the thyroid and may improve function in sinuses, throat, nasal passages, and eyes. In chronic headaches, the rolls may help if done often enough, three or four times daily.

LEG LIFT

Lie on back, place hands on the floor beside hips, palms down. Raise your head, bringing chin down to chest. Keeping body flat on floor, with legs absolutely straight, breathe in and slowly lift legs straight up over the head and slightly behind, pressing down on hands for leverage. Hold this posture for two or three seconds. Then, breathing out, bring legs, stiff-kneed, to the floor, and allow the head to drop gently back on the floor. Relax, and repeat this exercise two or three times to begin with, gradually working up to ten repetitions. The thyroid is again stimulated because of the chin action in the notch of the throat. With the legs raised, the pelvic organs are helpfully toned, and the muscles in the lower back and abdomen strengthened. By keeping the legs straight, muscles in the upper thighs stretch and become more flexible. In the beginning, if not able to bring the legs up straight, flex the knees, and bring the legs up in this fashion. Meanwhile, keep trying to do lift with the legs straight. In a week or so, as your muscles become stronger, you should manage. Repeat this exercise three times in the beginning, eventually working up to ten repetitions.

KNEE-BACK EXTENSION

This exercise from a kneeling position is designed to strengthen the pelvic area, and so enhance the virility, while giving a healthful stretch to the lower spine. It is a very simple exercise. Get on your knees, with your feet extended directly behind you, and your trunk erect. With your knees about a foot apart, breathing in lightly, reach both hands as far as you can behind the thighs, with the thumb hooked outside each thigh. Hands on thighs, lean body forward slightly, breathing out as your chin drops to the chest. And then, breathing in deeply, lean back from the hips, getting support from the hands. Arch the back slowly, and bring head back as far as it will comfortably go. Hold this backward extension for a couple of seconds. Then breathing out, and pressing hands against thighs, come forward, flexing from the waist and again bringing chin to chest as you reach center position. Remember to breathe only through the nostrils in the easy rhythm of the movements. Repeat the exercise three times and work up to ten repetitions.

This exercise is especially beneficial to the spine and the lower-back area, serving to stabilize an unstable sacro-iliac.

THE TABLE

The Upside-Down Body Lift is also known as the Table. In its hold position, the arms and legs, vertical to the floor serve as table-leg support for the body, stretched out at a tabletop level from head to knees.

Sit down with the trunk erect and the legs extended in front on the floor about a foot apart. Place both hands flat next to the hips, the fingertips backwards and even with the buttocks, or slightly back of buttocks, and just a little to the side. Bring the knees up from the floor and breathe in as you push up with arms and shoulders to bring the body to a horizontal position with the head straight back and level with the trunk. In this hold position, the legs and arms should be evenly perpendicular to the body, supporting it like the legs of a table. After holding for two or three seconds, relishing the relaxing stretch of the spine, lower the buttocks to the floor as you breathe out, and extend the legs, returning to the sitting position. Repeat this exercise two or three times in the beginning, always remembering that you extend your legs fully in front each time as a starting point.

This exercise strengthens arms and legs, the spine and abdominal muscles, the neck, and brings blood into the head, even as its up-and-down motion with the breathing improves the tone of the abdominal organs.

THE CAT

We call this the Cat exercise, as we alternately arch and hump the back as the cat does. It's a smart cat who does this exercise, as it may help make one of those nine lives enjoyable. As a cat does, you get on all fours with hands and knees about a foot apart. Arms and thighs are straight up and the head level with back. With palms pressed forward to floor and on toes, breathe in and lift buttocks up as high as you can, your body forming an inverted V. Hold this position for a second or two, humping the back, then breathing out with the head lowered, swing forward from straight arms, bringing the hips almost to the floor as the head goes up in the same motion. Repeat exercise three times if possible and build up to ten. Let the air in as you bring the body up, and out as you bring it down.

This exercise benefits nearly every area, particularly the lower back, and stresses co-ordination between body movement and breathing.

THE HEADSTAND

The Headstand is not for everyone, at least not in the beginning. But if you have come along with the other exercises, especially the Shoulder Stand, and are doing this easily, you are probably ready for the Headstand. While not essential to the routine, it does represent a certain achievement for the student, a sort of extra dividend. But don't feel dismayed if you never get to it, as the other exercises can keep you eternally youthful.

To begin, kneel down on a padded surface, a thick rug or mat, with a blanket folded four ways as an additional cushion. Then lower the head, establishing contact with the mat at the frontal hairline (or where it used to be), lightly interlocking your fingers around the head at the floor level. In this crouching position, bring the elbows in so that they are on a line with the knees, which are no more than a foot apart. All the weight is distributed along the arms and shoulders (not the head), which press solidly down. Do not allow elbows to fly out as this makes the exercise more difficult. With your forehead on the mat or floor, at the hairline, a good balancing point, and with your hands clasped around the head, you bring the buttocks up as high as you can while keeping straight legs extended as far back as you can comfortably. You are now ready to generate the momentum which will carry you to the top. On your toes, bending knees, take tiny steps forward, keeping the knees low, and the buttocks up. As the trunk becomes vertical with your forward motion, arch the back, scrunch on the elbows, putting all your weight there, tuck in the knees and then deliberately raise legs to the ceiling, remembering to arch the back and lean heavily on the elbows, which are on a line with the knees. Keep weight on elbows, breathing in and out easily through nose. As you practice this exercise, you will eventually find that it is possible to arch the back and balance from the hips in such a way that you can rest in this position weightlessly and effortlessly for five or ten minutes—though five minutes is sufficient to reverse the circulation and give the sagging abdominal organs a stimulating circulation change beneficial to the body's various natural functions.

Stay up no more than a few seconds the first time, bringing this to a minute in a week or so as you get used to the reverse flow of blood, and eventually five minutes as your balance improves. If unsure of your balance in the beginning, just bring yourself to the stage where you tuck in your legs. Eventually, bring your legs up at your pleasure. To come down from the Headstand, bend the knees and bring the legs down slowly, touching the floor with the toes. Then rise slowly from this kneeling position and rest.

THE CORRECTIVE EXERCISE

We repeat this exercise in conclusion because this is largely what the book is all about. The exercise is one hundred percent effective in bringing the sacroiliac joint back to its correct position if done properly. Pulling back the leg as you do this exercise is not as important as just holding the leg at the proper angle as it heels into the crotch. And in pulling back lightly and evenly on the leg with the hands on the ankle and behind the knee, the thrust is more outside than back. Even so there is not the slightest stress or strain. The angle is the thing.

Lying down, the left hand goes over the right ankle comfortably, and brings the heel near the groin. The right hand goes back and around the knee so that the fingers grasp the kneecap, with the heel as close to the crotch as you can manage. Hold this position for thirty to sixty seconds. Do not attempt to force the leg or yank it. Hold this angulated position in a relaxed way. Repeat with the other leg. You may also practice exercise in sitting and standing positions to facilitate resetting of sacroiliac at home, work, or play.

PEACE POSTURE

After completing the exercises lie on your back for five minutes, breathing in and out gently but deeply, mentally directing each muscle and joint to relax from head to toe. Then get up fresh and eager to carry on the day's activities. Think good thoughts and visualize pleasant scenes. Plunge into the day's activities and live them to the hilt. Live not only a long life but a joyous and productive one. That's what it's all about.

GLOSSARY OF FAMILIAR TERMS AS THEY RELATE TO THIS
BOOK

Adjustment—Manual manipulation of spine or other joints to relieve tension caused by their malposition or displacement.

Adrenals—The endocrine glands lying near or on the kidney which govern metabolism and which respond to physical and emotional emergencies.

Anterior—Front of any area, as the anterior sacroiliac ligaments or the anterior or frontal rotation of the ilium bone.

Apposition—Contact of two surfaces, as the sacrum and ilium correctly contacting each other.

Arrhythmia—An irregular beat of the heart.

Arteriosclerosis—Hardening of the arteries, brought on by the aging processes, usually marked by decreasing vascular circulation.

Arthritis—Inflammation of joints, marked by stiffening and calcium deposits.

Atrophy—A decrease in size or bulk of tissue, usually from disuse.

Autonomic—Automatic functions of the body, as in breathing, vascular circulation, heartbeat, digestion, all affected by the involuntary nervous system.

Bursitis—Inflammation of a saclike cavity, or bursa, which protectively lubricates a bony surface, such as a shoulder, elbow, or knee.

Cantilever—Usually a support projected from one end, as the flexed torso is supported from the sacroiliac. In animals, we have a double spinal cantilever, supported at both ends of the body.

Cartilage—A semi-hard, rubberlike connective tissue found throughout the body, supporting mobile joints, as in knee, jaw, and spine.

Cervical—Area of neck defined by seven cervical vertebrae.

Cholesterol—A white fatty crystalline substance found in bile, bloodstream, organs, and tissues. An excess may cause hardening of the arteries.

Chronic—A condition or disease of a fixed pattern and a long duration.

Coccyx—The tailbone consisting of four fused rudimentary vertebrae.

Compression—Forceful squeezing together of two surfaces, as the spinal discs being pressed down or flattened.

Condyle—The rounded surface at the head of a bone.

Corrective exercise—Self-help exercise designed to correct a displaced sacroiliac joint.

Crest—In the iliac crest, the outer and upper border of the ilial bone or hipbone.

Curvature—In the abnormal curvature of spine, as opposed to normal curvature, there is a lateral distortion of the spine, starting at the base of the spine and curving out on either side all the way up the base of the skull.

Declination—Drop of the iliac bone, or pelvis, as to cause a pelvic tilt.

Disc—A padlike, cushionlike, tough substance separating any two vertebrae.

Displacement—A radical change or misalignment of bones, ligaments, and tendons.

Dorsal—The twelve thoracic or dorsal vertebrae to which the ribs are attached.

Edema—Accumulation of fluid in tissues, often resulting from a traumatic strain or injury.

Electrolyte—Relating to a fluid interchange between cells of the body resulting in a flow of electrical energy indicating muscle performance.

Emesis—State of vomiting.

Emphysema—Disease of lung tissue limiting breathing capacity because of destructive changes in small bronchial tubes.

Encephalography—X-raying of brain, usually to determine presence of tumor.

Endocrine—The ductless glands, pituitary, thyroid, adrenals, and others, whose secretions pass directly into the bloodstream.

Estrogen—A hormone formed by the ovary in the female; its loss is usually associated with female change of life.

Eustachian tube—Tube from inner ear to nasal-pharynx tube balancing pressure in inner ear.

Femur—Long thigh bone.

Fibrous—Connective or fibrous tissue which forms in the process of healing.

Fusion—Surgical procedure to fuse two or more vertebrae together.

Gonads—Male and female sex glands, in testes and ovary.

Hormones—A stimulating internal secretion produced by the glands.

Hypertrophy—An overdevelopment of tissue from unusual stress.

Hyperthyroid—Excess activity of the thyroid gland tending one to nervousness and irritability.

Hypoglycemia—Rapid drop in blood sugar sometimes causing faintness and mental confusion.

Ilium—The hipbone attached to the sacrum to form the pelvis or sacroiliac joint.

Inflammation—Swelling and pain in tissue after an injury.

Innervation—Stimulation of nerve impulse.

Isometrics—A method of increasing muscle tone and strength by putting stress on the muscle without motion.

Laminectomy—Removal of the rear portion of one or more vertebrae.

Ligaments—Fibrous tissue connecting bone and cartilage and supporting muscle groups.

Lordosis—Abnormally exaggerated forward curvature of the lumbar spine.

Lumbar—Five vertebrae in the lower back above the sacrum.

Lymph—A nearly colorless fluid carrying white blood cells to the tissues.

Metabolism—The process by which the body assimilates food and oxygen and transforms it into useful energy and its byproducts.

Migraine—Agonizing headache usually on one side of head, generally accompanied by dizziness, nausea, sensitivity to light.

Muscle—A mass of soft tissue which expands and contracts to move the various parts of the skeleton.

Myelogram—X ray with use of dye to visualize spinal cord.

Myogram—Electrical test of the impulse of a nerve stimulus to a given muscle.

Nerve trunk—A cluster of nerves coming off the length of the spinal cord.

Ossicles—Tiny bones in inner ear conducting sound.

Otosclerosis—Hardening of the ossicles or tiny bones in the inner ear contributing to deafness.

Oxygenation—Combining of oxygen with red blood cells to increase strength and vitality.

Pelvis—The pelvic girdle, a bony saucerlike receptacle supporting the abdominal cavity, and composed of the hipbones, pubic bones, and coccyx.

Pituitary—The so-called master gland in the lower brain which helps to regulate growth, nutrition, metabolism.

Presbyopia—Middle-age vision in which muscle accommodation of near vision is reduced, as in reading or other close work.

Pubic bone—Two small bones which come together just above the crotch to form the front of the pelvic girdle.

Sacral plexus—A group of nerves coming out of the spinal cord at the lower end of the lumbar area and the upper sacrum area, and which affects the lower extremities.

Sacroiliac—The juncture of ilium or hipbone and the sacrum to form that joint which supports the weight of the entire trunk.

Sacrum—A V-shaped, slightly concave bone composed of five fused, immovable segments, attached by ligaments on either side to the hipbones.

Scapula—The shoulder blades, triangular flat, wingbones over the ribs and attached to each shoulder.

Sciatica—A nerve disorder often resulting from a sacroiliac displacement and marked by severe pains shooting down one or both legs.

Scoliosis—An abnormal lateral curvature of any section of the spinal column usually caused by a tilt of the pelvis.

Semicircular canals—Loop-shaped tubes which as part of the inner ear maintain the body's equilibrium.

Slippage—In sacroiliac slippage the ilium bone or hipbone slips from its normal position on the sacrum as a result of strain or stress.

Solar plexus—A group of nerves, largest of the autonomic nerve plexes, which is situated behind the stomach and sends nerve fibers to all of the abdominal organs.

Somatic—Relating to all bodily and organic functions that are generated automatically.

Spasm—Uncontrolled painful muscular contraction.

Sphincter—A round muscle anywhere in the body which contracts to close a tube or passage in the body.

Spinal cord—Thick longitudinal cord of nervous tissue protected by the vertebrae, extending from the base of the brain to the sacrum.

Spine—The vertebral column, including the vertebrae and the cord.

Spondylitis—Inflammation of one or more of the vertebrae.

Suboccipital bone—Bone at the base of the skull whose muscle attachments under stress become sensitive and instigate headaches.

Syncope—Sudden fall of blood pressure resulting in loss of consciousness.

Synovial fluid—A clear fluid acting as a lubricant in joints, bursae, and tendon surfaces.

Tendinitis—An inflammation of tendon resulting from strain.

Tendon—Fibrous cord connecting muscle to bony attachment and becoming part of the muscle movement.

Thyroid—Gland of internal secretion lying in the notch of the throat, whose function is essential to metabolic balance and proper growth of the body.

Tissue—An aggregate of cells which constitute in their varying nature the physical substance of the body.

Tone—A state of firmness or tension in body tissue, dependent on diet, exercise and circulation.

Toxic—An accumulation of poisonous wastes which in time can cause inflammation and illness.

Trauma—Damaging emotional or physical experience which shocks or injures any part of the body or mind.

Tuberosity—A knob, lump, or bump protruding from any part of the anatomy.

Tympanic membrane—Small nearly oval membrane closing externally the cavity of the inner ear and vibrating to sound waves to begin hearing process.

Varicose veins—Abnormally swollen or dilated veins caused by faulty circulation, usually in the legs.

Vascular—Relating to blood vessels and the blood.

Vasomotor—Nerve-power regulating the size of blood vessels.

Vertebra—A bony cylindrical segment of the spine, separated by discs. Twenty-four free-moving segments of vertebrae permit the spine to be flexible.

Whiplash—An injury generally received in a sitting position from a sudden blow which snaps back the neck and abruptly flexes the spine forward, then backward, resulting usually not only in damage to the neck and shoulders but to the spine as well.

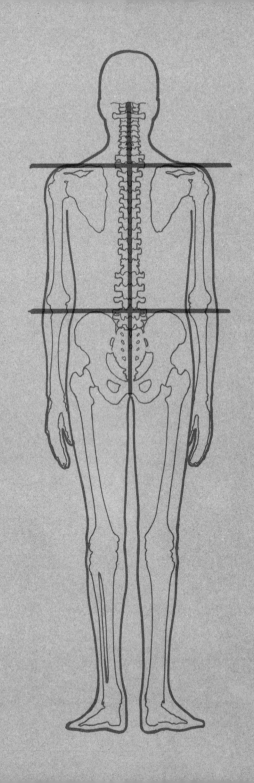